STOP MASSAGE !

Instead Fix Your Atlas Bone

Heal Yourself by Correcting the First Cervical Vertebra: C1

Top 25 Specialists Worldwide

To Rebirth

© Christophe Paroni - 2024

TABLE OF CONTENT

Description Atlas Bone   p.9

Introduction   p.11

The Atlas Bone: The Missing Key to Health

- Overview of the Atlas vertebra and its significance.
- Personal anecdotes or testimonies from people who have benefited from Atlas adjustments.
- Mention of the potential connection between Atlas misalignment and symptoms such as tension, nerve pain, heart palpitations, migraines, dizziness, fatigue, and overall body imbalance.
- Brief historical background on the discovery and importance of the Atlas bone's role in health.

Chapter 1:   p.15

Understanding the Atlas: The First Cervical Vertebra

- Detailed explanation of the anatomical structure and function of the Atlas vertebra.
- The relationship between the Atlas, the spine, and the nervous system.
- How Atlas misalignment can create widespread tension and dysfunction in the body.
- Why traditional medical treatments often miss the Atlas's role in chronic health conditions.

Chapter 2: p.21

How Atlas Misalignment Affects the Body

- Common physical symptoms: headaches, neck pain, migraines, dizziness, vision issues, and musculoskeletal problems.
- Nervous system effects: nerve compression, neuralgia, stress on the vagus nerve, and autonomic dysfunction.
- Emotional and mental health: anxiety, insomnia, and cognitive impairments linked to Atlas dysfunction.
- Detailed discussion on how Atlas misalignment impacts posture, causing compensation patterns throughout the body.
- Case studies of people who have experienced profound health changes after correcting their Atlas.

Chapter 3: p.37

The Art and Science of Atlas Adjustment

- Overview of the science behind Atlas adjustment and its effects on the central nervous system.
- Different methods of Atlas correction (manual techniques vs. instruments).
- Detailed explanation of Atlas Orthogonal Technique, a precise, non-invasive adjustment method using specialized instruments.
    - Mention practitioners like Dr. Roy Sweat, the founder of Atlas Orthogonal Chiropractic.
- How technology has improved these techniques over the last few decades.

Chapter 4: p.47

Self-Regulation and Regeneration: How to Heal Yourself

- Techniques and exercises that help maintain Atlas alignment at home.
- Understanding how posture, ergonomics, and movement patterns can influence Atlas stability.
- Breathing exercises and meditation to reduce nervous system tension that affects the Atlas.
- Healing practices for regeneration: nutritional advice, physical therapy, and gentle stretching.
- Tools and aids such as pillows, braces, or supports that can assist in keeping the Atlas in position.

Chapter 5: p.59

Atlas Healing: A Global Phenomenon

- Profiles of renowned Atlas healers around the world.
    - **USA**: Introduction to Dr. Jeff McGuckin, a leading Atlas practitioner in the United States who has developed his unique approach.
    - **Canada**: Highlight **Dr. Dennis Poole**, who uses state-of-the-art techniques in Toronto to treat Atlas misalignments.
    - **Switzerland**: Profile **Yves Humbert**, a prominent Atlas healer who has worked with a 20-year-old machine passed down from his teacher in Sion, Switzerland.
- Description of their methods, philosophies, and success stories from patients.

Chapter 6: p.75

Atlas Joint Instability: Causes, Consequences, and Solutions

- A deep dive into Atlas joint instability, its causes (e.g., trauma, poor posture, stress), and how it develops.
- The consequences of long-term Atlas instability on overall health.
- Effective solutions for stabilizing the Atlas and preventing further misalignments.
- Techniques that focus on restoring proper movement to the head, neck, and spine.

Chapter 7: p.87

A Second Rebirth: Stories of Healing and Transformation

- Real-life stories of people who have experienced what feels like a second rebirth after having their Atlas adjusted.
- Examples of improved movement, reduced pain, and the restoration of balance in their lives.
- Testimonials of patients from across the globe who have gone through different healing methods, including those who sought help from traditional healers and those who used high-tech Atlas adjustment devices.
- How Atlas correction has changed people's quality of life, including chronic illness remission, improved posture, and emotional well-being.

Chapter 8: p.97

How to Find and Work with an Atlas Specialist

- Practical advice on how to find a certified and skilled Atlas specialist.

- What to expect during your first visit and ongoing treatment.
- Questions to ask when selecting a practitioner.
- Resources for Atlas care in various countries (directories of practitioners and clinics).

Chapter 9: p.113

The Future of Atlas Therapy: Cutting-Edge Research and Innovations

- A look at ongoing research in the field of Atlas therapy and spinal health.
- The role of technology in improving accuracy and efficacy in treatments.
- Potential future applications, including wearable technology that can monitor and support Atlas alignment.
- How the growing awareness of Atlas misalignment is impacting the medical and wellness communities.

Conclusion: p.121

Healing from the Inside Out:
Reiterate the life-changing potential of addressing Atlas misalignment.

Appendices: p.124

- **Appendix A**: Practitioner Directories

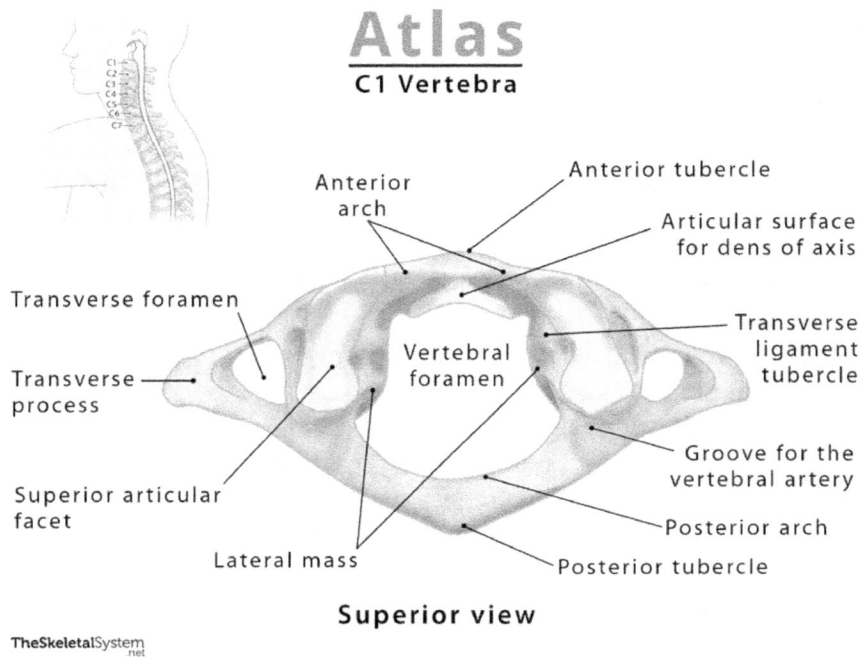

Source : The Skeleta System

Description of the Atlas Bone (C1 Vertebra)

The **Atlas bone, or C1 vertebra**, (see left image) is the first cervical vertebra at the top of the spine, directly supporting the skull. Here are the key features:

1. **Anterior Arch**: This is the front portion of the Atlas. It is a thin, curved part of the bone that provides attachment points for ligaments and muscles.

2. **Posterior Arch**: This is the back part of the Atlas, broader and more substantial than the anterior arch. It provides protection to the spinal cord.

3. **Transverse Processes**: These are the wing-like projections on either side of the Atlas. They serve as attachment points for muscles and ligaments.

4. **Vertebral Foramen**: The large central hole through which the spinal cord passes.

5. **Superior Articular Facets**: Located on the top of the Atlas, these are concave surfaces that articulate with the occipital condyles of the skull, allowing for the nodding motion of the head.

6. **Inferior Articular Facets**: Located on the bottom of the Atlas, these articulate with the second cervical vertebra (Axis or C2), enabling rotational movement of the head.

7. **Transverse Foramina**: Holes in the transverse processes through which the vertebral artery and vein pass.

"Three or four times a day, you need to relax when you're at the computer. You need to walk, relax, and consciously focus on relaxing your body. All the muscles are tense around the joints." —

Yves Humbert, Atlas Healer in Europe

Introduction: The Atlas Bone:
The Missing Key to Health

The human body is a marvel of engineering, with each component intricately connected to the next. Among the most crucial yet often overlooked elements is the Atlas bone, or the first cervical vertebra called (**C1**). The bone is named for Atlas of Greek mythology, just as Atlas bore the weight of the heavens, the first cervical vertebra supports the head. [1]This small, ring-like bone plays a pivotal role in supporting the skull, facilitating movement, and protecting the spinal cord.

However, when the Atlas is misaligned, it can cause a cascade of health issues, including chronic pain, nerve dysfunction, and even emotional and cognitive disturbances.

Most people seek relief through osteopathy, massages, or physical therapy because their neck feels blocked or tense. While these treatments may provide temporary relief, they do not address the root cause of the problem. In many cases, the underlying issue is a misaligned Atlas. Some individuals experience such intense tension that they end up consulting a cardiologist for heart palpitations, only to be prescribed medication that doesn't resolve the issue. Nothing seems to work because the real culprit lies in a single vertebra—the Atlas.

When the Atlas is out of alignment, it disrupts the balance of the entire body, leading to various health problems. The solution is to correct the alignment of the Atlas, which can bring remarkable changes in overall health and well-being. This book will help you discover what the Atlas is, how to realign it, and, most importantly, which specialists to contact for help—whether in the USA, Africa, Latin America, or Europe.

---

[1] *Source : Wikipedia https://en.wikipedia.org/wiki/Atlas_(anatomy)*

The directory of specialists can be found at the end of the book to guide you in your journey toward better health. By the time you finish reading, you will have gained the knowledge needed to take control of your health and experience a rebirth of sorts—a chance to restore balance and vitality to your body.

*" Welcome to a new life beginning.
When I finished my first Session with the practitioner,
it was like a rebirth ."*

Angela

Chapter 1: Understanding the Atlas:

The First Cervical Vertebra

"The foundation of wellness starts at the top."

The human body is a complex, **interconnected system** where every part has a role to play in maintaining balance and health. Yet, when we think about wellness, how often do we consider the bones in our neck? Never ! Period. The truth is, we should be thinking about them all the time — especially about one in particular: the Atlas bone.

What is the Atlas Bone?

The Atlas bone, scientifically known as the C1 vertebra, is the first cervical vertebra located at the very top of the spine, as mow you know it. Its name comes from the Greek myth of Atlas, the Titan condemned to hold up the sky for eternity. Much like its mythological namesake, the Atlas bone holds up the head, supporting the skull's weight and facilitating a wide range of movements, or not.

- **Anatomy of the Atlas**: The Atlas is unique among the vertebrae. Unlike the other vertebrae in your spine, it doesn't have a body or a spinous process (the bony projection you can feel along your back). Instead, it's more of a ring-like structure with a large central hole — the vertebral foramen — through which the spinal cord passes. This design allows for the extensive range of motion in the neck, including nodding and rotating your head.

- **Superior and Inferior Articular Facets**: The Atlas has two concave, kidney-shaped areas on its top surface known as the superior articular facets. These facets cradle the occipital condyles of the skull, allowing the head to nod in a "yes" motion. On the bottom of the Atlas, the inferior articular facets connect with the second cervical vertebra, the axis (C2), which enables the "no" rotational movement of the head.

- **Transverse Processes and Foramina**: The Atlas has transverse processes extending outwards on each side, which serve as attachment points for muscles and ligaments. Each process has a hole called the transverse foramen, through which the vertebral artery and vein travel, supplying blood to the brain.

The Atlas's Crucial Role in Health

The Atlas's position and function make it one of the most important bones in the body, despite its small size. It is the pivotal point for nearly every movement of the head, and its alignment directly influences the entire spine. Here's why this matters:

- **Support and Movement**: The Atlas not only supports the skull but also facilitates the head's range of motion. Imagine trying to balance a bowling ball on a ring—this is essentially what your Atlas is doing every day, and it needs to be perfectly aligned to function correctly.

- **Protection of the Spinal Cord**: The Atlas acts as a protective ring around the spinal cord, especially as it transitions from the brainstem. Any misalignment here can result in pressure on the spinal cord or the brainstem, leading to a variety of neurological symptoms, including headaches, dizziness, and even systemic issues like high blood pressure.

- **The Gateway to the Nervous System**: The nervous system is the body's command center, controlling everything from muscle movements to hormone release. The Atlas's alignment is crucial because even a slight misalignment can disrupt the nervous system's communication pathways. This disruption can manifest as pain, impaired mobility, or dysfunction in other parts of the body.

The Domino Effect of Atlas Misalignment

"Fix the head, and the body will follow." This adage is particularly true when it comes to the Atlas bone. When the Atlas is out of alignment, the effects can be felt throughout the entire body, creating a domino effect of problems.

- **Postural Imbalance**: The body's instinct is to keep the eyes level with the horizon. When the Atlas is misaligned, the head tilts, causing the rest of the spine to compensate. This compensation leads to a chain reaction down the entire spinal column, resulting in poor posture, back pain, and even hip or knee issues.

- **Nerve Impingement**: A misaligned Atlas can press against the spinal cord or nearby nerves, leading to a variety of symptoms such as tingling, numbness, or chronic pain. This impingement can also affect the autonomic nervous system, which controls involuntary functions like heart rate, digestion, and breathing.

- **Blood Flow Restriction**: The vertebral arteries pass through the transverse foramina of the Atlas to supply blood to the brain. If the Atlas is misaligned, it can restrict this blood flow, leading to symptoms such as headaches, dizziness, and even cognitive issues like brain fog.

An Ancient Problem with Modern Solutions

The concept of the Atlas bone and its significance is not new. Ancient practices like yoga and traditional chiropractic methods have long emphasized the importance of **spinal alignment**. However, the modern understanding of the Atlas's role has been significantly enhanced by advanced technology and research.

- **Historical Perspective**: Hippocrates, often called the "*Father of Medicine,*" recognized the importance of spinal health. He famously said, **"Look well to the spine for the cause of disease."** The Atlas, as the topmost vertebra, was understood even then as a <u>key player in maintaining overall health</u>.

- **Modern Research**: Recent studies have reinforced the Atlas's significance in health. A study published in the *Journal of Upper Cervical Chiropractic Research* found that realignment of the Atlas vertebra could lead to significant reductions in blood pressure among patients with hypertension . Another study highlighted in *Frontiers in Neurology* emphasized how misalignment can lead to impaired cerebral blood flow, which is linked to migraines and other neurological conditions .

Understanding Your Atlas: The First Step to Healing

Awareness of the Atlas bone is the first step in addressing many chronic health issues that may have been incorrectly attributed to other causes. It's not just about neck pain—it's about your entire body's well-being.

- **The Atlas as the Body's Foundation**: Think of your Atlas as the foundation of a house. If the foundation is off, the walls, floors, and roof will be unstable. Correcting your Atlas alignment can bring stability and balance to your entire body, improving both physical and neurological health.

- **A Simple Adjustment with Profound Effects**: Despite its complexity, the process of correcting an Atlas misalignment is often surprisingly simple and non-invasive. Techniques like the Atlas Orthogonal method or NUCCA (National Upper Cervical Chiropractic Association) care involve precise adjustments that can result in immediate relief and long-term health benefits.

Conclusion: The Atlas — Your Body's Best-Kept Secret

Understanding the Atlas bone and its impact on your health is like discovering the missing piece of a puzzle. For many, addressing this small but mighty bone is the key to unlocking a future free of pain, full of energy, and brimming with vitality.

As we move through the following chapters, we'll explore the many ways in which the Atlas affects your health, how to diagnose misalignment, and the different methods available to correct it. Remember, the foundation of wellness starts at the top, and by fixing your Atlas, you can set the stage for a healthier, happier life.

References:

1. *Groch, M. W., & Browning, T. E. (2007). Atlas vertebra realignment and the reduction of arterial blood pressure: a pilot study. Journal of Upper Cervical Chiropractic Research. Retrieved from uppercervicalsubluxation.com*

2. *Damasceno, D. D., & Lima, M. F. (2019). Atlas misalignment and cerebral blood flow: the connection to migraines. Frontiers in Neurology. Retrieved from frontiersin.org*

Chapter 2: How Atlas Misalignment Affects the Body

"The Atlas may be small, but its impact is monumental."

The human body is an intricately connected system, where even the slightest imbalance can send shockwaves through your entire being. When it comes to the Atlas bone, this statement couldn't be more accurate. The Atlas, as the first cervical vertebra, plays a pivotal role in supporting the head and facilitating communication between the brain and body. When the Atlas is misaligned, it can disrupt this delicate balance, leading to a wide range of health issues that are often misdiagnosed or treated symptomatically without addressing the root cause.

Physical Symptoms of Atlas Misalignment

"Wherever the Atlas goes, the body follows."

One of the most immediate and noticeable effects of an Atlas misalignment is physical discomfort, particularly in the neck, head, and upper back. However, the scope of physical symptoms can be much broader and more complex...

- **Neck Pain and Stiffness**: The most common symptom of Atlas misalignment is neck pain, often accompanied by stiffness and restricted movement. Because the Atlas supports the skull, any deviation from its proper position can create tension and strain in the surrounding muscles and ligaments. This can lead to chronic neck pain that is difficult to relieve through traditional methods like massage or physical therapy.

- **Headaches and Migraines**: Many people who suffer from frequent headaches or migraines may be experiencing the consequences of an Atlas misalignment. The tension caused by the misalignment can radiate up into the head, resulting in pressure headaches. Additionally, as we'll explore later, an

Atlas misalignment can affect blood flow to the brain, which is a known trigger for migraines.

- **Shoulder and Back Pain**: When the Atlas is out of alignment, the entire spine compensates, leading to a cascading effect that can cause pain in the shoulders, upper back, and even the lower back. This is because the muscles and ligaments work harder to keep the head balanced, creating tension and discomfort in other parts of the body.

- **Jaw Pain and TMJ Disorders**: The jaw is closely connected to the Atlas bone through the temporomandibular joint (TMJ). Misalignment of the Atlas can cause the jaw to shift out of its natural position, leading to TMJ disorders, which are characterized by jaw pain, clicking, and difficulty chewing.

Nervous System Disruption

"The Atlas is the gatekeeper of the nervous system."

The Atlas bone is not just responsible for supporting the head; it also plays a crucial role in protecting the nervous system. The spinal cord, which carries messages between the brain and the rest of the body, passes through the Atlas. When the Atlas is misaligned, it can compress or irritate the spinal cord and nearby nerves, leading to a variety of neurological symptoms and pains.

- **Nerve Compression and Radiating Pain**: A misaligned Atlas can press against nerves, particularly those in the upper cervical spine. This can result in radiating pain that extends into the arms and hands, often mistaken for conditions like carpal tunnel syndrome. Patients may experience tingling, numbness, or a burning sensation along the nerve pathways.

- **Autonomic Nervous System Dysfunction**: The autonomic nervous system (**ANS**) controls involuntary functions like heart rate, digestion, and breathing. The Atlas's proximity to the brainstem means that its misalignment can interfere with the ANS, leading to symptoms such as heart palpitations, irregular heartbeat, digestive issues, and respiratory problems. This disruption can also contribute to conditions like chronic fatigue syndrome and fibromyalgia.

- **Vagus Nerve Impairment**: The vagus nerve, one of the longest nerves in the body, runs close to the Atlas. It plays a significant role in regulating the parasympathetic nervous system, which controls rest and digestion. Misalignment of the Atlas can irritate the vagus nerve, leading to symptoms such as nausea, **acid reflux**, and an inability to relax or sleep well.

The Emotional and Cognitive Impact of the C1

"When the Atlas is out of place, so is your peace of mind."

The effects of an Atlas misalignment are not confined to the physical body; they can also extend to your emotional and mental well-being. Because the Atlas influences blood flow to the brain and the functioning of the nervous system, its misalignment can contribute to a variety of cognitive and emotional disturbances.

- **Anxiety and Depression**: Many people with an Atlas misalignment report feelings of anxiety and depression. This is partly due to the physical discomfort and pain associated with the misalignment, which can wear down your emotional resilience. Moreover, disruptions in the autonomic nervous system can exacerbate these feelings, as the body is constantly in a state of stress or fight-or-flight.

- **Cognitive Impairments**: A misaligned Atlas can reduce blood flow to the brain, particularly to the areas responsible for memory, concentration, and executive function. This can result in brain fog, memory lapses, and difficulty focusing on tasks. These symptoms are often mistaken for the normal effects of aging or stress, but they may actually be linked to Atlas dysfunction.

- **Sleep Disorders**: The Atlas's influence on the nervous system and blood flow can also affect sleep quality. People with a misaligned Atlas often struggle with insomnia or poor-quality sleep, as their bodies are unable to fully relax. This lack of restorative sleep can lead to a vicious cycle of fatigue, irritability, and further emotional distress.

The Domino Effect:
How One Small Bone Can Create Big Problems

"A misaligned Atlas is like a crooked keystone in an arch; everything around it begins to crumble."

The body is **THE master of compensation.** When something is out of balance, other parts of the body adjust to maintain stability.

However, these compensatory mechanisms can lead to further problems, creating a domino effect of symptoms that may seem unrelated but are, in fact, connected to the misalignment of the Atlas.

- **Postural Distortions**: When the Atlas is misaligned, the body adjusts to keep the eyes level with the horizon. This often results in a tilted head, uneven shoulders, and a curved spine. Over time, these postural distortions can lead to chronic pain and musculoskeletal issues that extend well beyond the neck and head.

- **Degenerative Changes**: Chronic misalignment of the Atlas can accelerate wear and tear on the spine and joints. As the body struggles to compensate for the misalignment, it places additional stress on the vertebrae, leading to degenerative changes such as osteoarthritis, herniated discs, and spinal stenosis.

- **Visceral Issues**: The effects of an Atlas misalignment can even extend to the body's internal organs. The nervous system's disruption can affect the function of the heart, lungs, and digestive system, contributing to issues such as high blood pressure, asthma, and irritable bowel syndrome.

Misdiagnosis and the Failure of Traditional Treatments

"Treating the symptoms without addressing the cause is like putting a band-aid on a bullet wound."

One of the most frustrating aspects of Atlas misalignment is how often it is overlooked or misdiagnosed due to lack of awareness. Many patients spend years treating the symptoms—**whether it's chronic pain, anxiety, blocked nerves in the neck, tension, or digestive issues**—without ever identifying the Atlas as the root cause.

Orthopedic Treatments: Patients with Atlas misalignment often seek help from orthopedic specialists for neck or back pain. Most commonly, this results in decades of treatments without any long-term results. While these treatments can provide temporary relief, they rarely address the underlying misalignment, leading to continued discomfort.

Massage Therapy: Massage can help alleviate muscle tension and pain associated with Atlas misalignment, but without correcting the misalignment itself, the relief is usually short-lived. After 2-3 days, the pain returns, and suddenly, you find yourself becoming a lifelong client of the medical system.

Medications: Many people with Atlas misalignment are prescribed medications for pain, anxiety, or digestive issues. However, these drugs only mask the symptoms without addressing the root problem, leading to dependency and possible side effects. Welcome to the world of chronic pain and antidepressants—an enormous market in which you become a permanent customer.

A Holistic Approach: The Importance of Addressing Atlas Misalignment

"Healing starts at the source."

The key to overcoming the wide-ranging effects of Atlas misalignment is to address the root cause, rather than just the symptoms. By focusing on realigning the Atlas, you can restore balance to your body, allowing it to heal naturally and more effectively.

- **Atlas Orthogonal and NUCCA Care**: These specialized chiropractic techniques focus on precisely realigning the Atlas, using gentle and non-invasive methods. Patients often experience <u>immediate relief from symptom</u>s, followed by a gradual improvement in overall health as the body begins to recover from the effects of the misalignment.

- **Complementary Therapies**: In addition to Atlas correction, complementary therapies such as physical therapy, acupuncture, and yoga can help support the healing process by strengthening the muscles, improving posture, and reducing stress.

- **Lifestyle Adjustments**: Maintaining Atlas alignment requires a holistic approach that includes proper posture, regular exercise, and stress management. By making these lifestyle changes, you can support the health of your Atlas and prevent future misalignments.

Conclusion: The Atlas as the Key to Total Wellness

The effects of an Atlas misalignment are far-reaching, affecting everything from physical comfort to mental clarity and emotional balance. Understanding the critical role of the Atlas in your overall health is the first step toward addressing chronic issues that may have been misdiagnosed or overlooked.

Chapter 2: How Atlas Misalignment Affects the Body (Continued)

The Far-Reaching Consequences of Ignoring Atlas Misalignment

"The body speaks in whispers before it screams."

It's not uncommon for people to endure years of unexplained symptoms, often **bouncing between specialists** who treat the symptoms but never quite solve the underlying issue. The problem with ignoring Atlas misalignment is that the body will continue to compensate, creating deeper and more complex health issues over time. This section will explore the long-term consequences of untreated Atlas misalignment and emphasize the importance of early intervention.

Chronic Pain and Fatigue

When the Atlas is misaligned, the muscles surrounding the neck and shoulders often become tight and overworked. Over time, this constant state of tension can lead to chronic pain conditions like fibromyalgia, where the body becomes hypersensitive to pain. What starts as occasional discomfort can evolve into a debilitating condition that affects every aspect of life.

- **The Pain Cycle**: Chronic pain often leads to fatigue, as the body expends extra energy trying to cope with the discomfort. This fatigue, in turn, can exacerbate the pain, creating a vicious cycle that is difficult to break. Many people with Atlas misalignment find themselves trapped in this cycle, seeking relief through pain medications, which only offer temporary respite.

- **Impact on Daily Life**: The combination of chronic pain and fatigue can have a significant impact on daily life. Activities that were once simple, like walking, sitting at a desk, or even sleeping, can become challenging. This can lead to a decrease in physical activity, which further weakens the body and perpetuates the cycle of pain and fatigue.

Systemic Health Issues

As the body struggles to maintain balance with a misaligned Atlas, other systems may begin to suffer. The ripple effect can lead to systemic health issues that seem unrelated at first glance but are actually connected to the underlying spinal misalignment.

- **Cardiovascular Problems**: The nervous system's disruption due to Atlas misalignment can extend to the cardiovascular system. Studies have shown that realigning the Atlas can lead to a significant reduction in high blood pressure. This is because the misaligned Atlas can exert pressure on the brainstem, which controls blood pressure regulation. Persistent misalignment may contribute to chronic hypertension, increasing the risk of heart disease and stroke.

- **Respiratory Issues**: Some individuals with Atlas misalignment experience breathing difficulties, such as shortness of breath or a feeling of constriction in the chest. This can be due to the effect of the misalignment on the vagus nerve, which influences the parasympathetic nervous system and controls the lungs. **Restoring Atlas alignment can relieve this pressure, improving respiratory function and reducing symptoms like asthma or chronic bronchitis**.

- **Digestive Disorders**: The connection between the spine and the digestive system is well-established, with the nervous system playing a crucial role in digestion. A misaligned Atlas can disrupt the signals between the brain and the digestive organs, leading to conditions such as acid reflux, constipation, and irritable bowel syndrome (IBS). Many patients report significant improvements in their digestive health after correcting Atlas misalignment.

Mental Health and Cognitive Decline

The impact of Atlas misalignment on mental health and cognitive function cannot be overstated. The brain requires a steady supply of oxygen and nutrients, which are delivered through the blood vessels passing through the cervical spine. When the Atlas is out of place, this blood flow can be compromised, leading to a range of cognitive and emotional disturbances.

- **Brain Fog and Memory Issues**: Reduced blood flow to the brain, particularly to the prefrontal cortex, can result in brain fog, characterized by confusion, forgetfulness, and difficulty concentrating. Over time, this can impair memory and the ability to make decisions, affecting both personal and professional life.

- **Anxiety and Mood Disorders**: The physical discomfort and neurological disruption caused by Atlas misalignment can contribute to anxiety and mood disorders. Chronic pain and the stress of dealing with ongoing health issues can lead to feelings of hopelessness, depression, and irritability. Moreover, the body's inability to properly relax due to nervous system imbalances can exacerbate these emotional states.

- **Cognitive Decline**: In more severe cases, untreated Atlas misalignment can contribute to long-term cognitive decline. The constant strain on the nervous system and reduced cerebral blood flow can increase the risk of developing neurodegenerative conditions like Alzheimer's disease and dementia.

Real-Life Case Studies: The Hidden Atlas Connection

"Sometimes the smallest things can have the biggest impact."

To bring these concepts to life, let's explore some real-life case studies of individuals who suffered from a range of chronic conditions—only to discover that their Atlas misalignment was the hidden cause.

Case Study 1: The Unresolved Migraine

- **Background**: Jane, a 35-year-old marketing executive, had been suffering from debilitating migraines for over a decade. Despite visiting multiple neurologists and trying various treatments, including medication and lifestyle changes, nothing provided lasting relief.

- **The Atlas Connection**: After a chance referral to an upper cervical chiropractor, Jane learned about the possible connection between her migraines and Atlas misalignment. A series of X-rays confirmed that her Atlas was indeed out of alignment.

- **Outcome**: After just a few sessions of Atlas correction, Jane noticed a significant reduction in the frequency and intensity of her migraines. Within six months, her migraines had nearly disappeared, and she was able to stop taking her medication entirely.

Case Study 2: The Chronic Fatigue Mystery

- **Background**: David, a 42-year-old teacher, struggled with chronic fatigue and persistent back pain that had worsened over the years. He tried physical therapy, dietary changes, and various supplements, but nothing seemed to help.

- **The Atlas Connection**: A friend recommended that David see a chiropractor who specialized in the Atlas Orthogonal technique. After an initial assessment, it was clear that David's Atlas was significantly misaligned, leading to widespread tension and stress on his body.

- **Outcome**: Following a series of Atlas adjustments, David's energy levels began to improve. His back pain also decreased as his posture improved and his body started to recover from years of compensating for the misalignment. Over time, David was able to return to his active lifestyle, feeling more vibrant and pain-free than he had in years.

Case Study 3: The Heart Palpitations

Background: Angela, a 44-year-old executive living in Switzerland, had been experiencing frequent heart palpitations and anxiety. Multiple tests ruled out any serious heart conditions, but the palpitations persisted, leaving her feeling anxious and unwell.

The Atlas Connection: Angela's chiropractor didn't suggest anything, but a friend told her about a method used in Valais, a mountainous region of Switzerland, where a certain healer was helping people by adjusting the Atlas. After seeing countless specialists with no results, she never would have thought her palpitations were related to her Atlas. After just two sessions with a specialist (see the list at the end of this book), her symptoms disappeared, including the palpitations — without any medication.

- **Outcome**: After undergoing a series of 2 Atlas adjustments, Angela's palpitations stopped. Her anxiety also improved, as the adjustments helped to regulate her autonomic nervous system, bringing her body back into balance, *"like a baby"*, she said.

Moving Toward a Solution: The Importance of Early Diagnosis

"A problem well diagnosed is a problem half solved."

The stories shared above highlight the transformative potential of addressing Atlas misalignment. However, the key to unlocking these benefits lies in early diagnosis and treatment. Many of the conditions associated with Atlas misalignment are progressive, meaning they can worsen over time if left uncorrected. Therefore, it's crucial to recognize the signs and symptoms of Atlas misalignment early on and seek out appropriate care.

- **Diagnostic Tools**: Advances in medical imaging have made it easier than ever to diagnose Atlas misalignment. Digital X-rays, CT scans, and MRIs can provide detailed images of the cervical spine, allowing practitioners to identify even subtle misalignments that might be contributing to health issues.

- **Screening and Self-Assessment**: While professional diagnosis is essential, there are also simple self-assessment techniques that can help individuals identify potential Atlas misalignment. These might include checking for uneven shoulder heights, persistent neck pain, or recurring headaches.

- **Seeking Professional Help**: If you suspect that you might have an Atlas misalignment, it's important to seek out a qualified healthcare provider who specializes in upper cervical care. Whether through chiropractic, osteopathy, or other forms of treatment, addressing the misalignment can lead to significant improvements in your overall health. **<u>Certain specialists are capable of detecting the position of the Atlas with their fingers and determining whether it is correctly aligned.</u>**

Conclusion: The Atlas as a Hidden Catalyst of Health

The Atlas bone, though small, plays a monumental role in the body's overall function. **Its alignment is critical not just for physical comfort, but for the proper functioning of the nervous system, circulation, and even mental well-being.** When the Atlas is misaligned, the ripple effects can lead to a wide range of health issues, many of which are misdiagnosed or inadequately treated because the true cause is overlooked.

Understanding the role of the Atlas in your health is the first step toward regaining control of your well-being. By addressing this often-hidden cause of chronic health problems, you can experience relief, restoration, and a renewed sense of vitality. In the next chapter, we will explore the various techniques and methods used to diagnose and correct Atlas misalignment, and how these approaches can help you achieve lasting health and wellness.

Chapter 3: The Art and Science of Atlas Adjustment

"Correct the foundation, and the structure will follow."

In the previous chapters, we've explored the crucial role of the Atlas bone in overall health and the wide range of symptoms that can result from its misalignment. Now, it's time to delve into the methods used to diagnose and correct Atlas misalignment. This chapter will guide you through the art and science of Atlas adjustment, from cutting-edge techniques to the holistic approaches that have helped countless people regain their health.

The Challenge of Atlas Diagnosis

"Not everything that counts can be counted, and not everything that can be counted counts." — *Albert Einstein*

Diagnosing Atlas misalignment is both an art and a science. While advanced imaging technology provides clear pictures of the spine's alignment, the real skill lies in interpreting these images and understanding how a subtle misalignment might be affecting the body's overall function. Let's explore the methods practitioners use to diagnose Atlas misalignment accurately, when use rays.

- **Advanced Imaging Techniques**: The most reliable way to diagnose Atlas misalignment is through advanced imaging techniques. Digital X-rays, CT scans, and MRIs offer detailed views of the cervical spine, allowing practitioners to see the exact position of the Atlas bone in relation to the skull and other cervical vertebrae. These images help to identify even minute deviations from the ideal alignment, which could be the root cause of a patient's symptoms.

- **Functional Assessments**: Beyond imaging, many practitioners use functional assessments to evaluate how Atlas misalignment is affecting the body. These assessments might include posture analysis, gait analysis, and neurological exams that test reflexes, muscle strength, and range of motion. By observing how the body moves and responds, practitioners can gain insights into the extent of the misalignment and its impact on the nervous system.

- **Patient History and Symptoms**: A thorough patient history is essential for accurate diagnosis. Practitioners often spend significant time discussing a patient's symptoms, lifestyle, and health history to understand how the Atlas misalignment developed and how it might be contributing to current health issues. This holistic approach ensures that the treatment plan addresses not just the symptoms, but the underlying causes as well.

Atlas Orthogonal Technique: Precision Meets Care

"Gentle yet powerful—that's the essence of the Atlas Orthogonal technique."

The Atlas Orthogonal (AO) technique is one of the most precise and non-invasive methods for correcting Atlas misalignment. Developed by Dr. Roy Sweat in the 1960s, this technique has helped thousands of people find relief from chronic pain, neurological issues, and other health problems related to Atlas misalignment.

- **How It Works**: The AO technique uses a specialized instrument to deliver a precise, gentle adjustment to the Atlas bone. Unlike traditional chiropractic methods that involve manual manipulation, the AO instrument is designed to apply a controlled force based on the specific measurements of the patient's misalignment. This precision ensures that the Atlas is moved back into its correct position without causing any undue strain or discomfort.

- **The Role of X-Rays**: Before performing an adjustment, practitioners using the AO technique typically take a series of X-rays to determine the exact nature of the misalignment. These images are analyzed using mathematical calculations to guide the adjustment process. By understanding the angle and direction of the misalignment, practitioners can tailor the adjustment to the patient's unique needs, ensuring maximum effectiveness.

- **Patient Experience**: One of the key benefits of the AO technique is its gentle nature. Patients often describe the adjustment as feeling like a light tap, with no discomfort or pain during the procedure. Despite the subtlety of the adjustment, the results can be profound, with many patients experiencing immediate relief from symptoms like headaches, neck pain, and dizziness.

- **Scientific Support**: The AO technique is backed by research showing its effectiveness in reducing symptoms associated with Atlas misalignment. Studies have demonstrated significant improvements in conditions like hypertension, migraines, and even lower back pain following AO adjustments. This evidence underscores the importance of precise, targeted care in addressing the root causes of health problems.

NUCCA: A Gentle Approach to Atlas Correction

"Alignment is everything."

The *National Upper Cervical Chiropractic Association* (NUCCA) offers another highly respected approach to Atlas correction. Founded in the 1960s, NUCCA focuses on gentle, non-invasive adjustments that are tailored to each patient's specific misalignment. The goal of NUCCA care is to restore the body's natural alignment and allow the nervous system to function optimally.

- **NUCCA Philosophy**: The NUCCA approach is based on the principle that proper spinal alignment is essential for overall health. When the spine is aligned, the nervous system can communicate effectively with the rest of the body, leading to better function and reduced symptoms. NUCCA practitioners aim to correct the Atlas misalignment in a way that minimizes the need for repeated adjustments, allowing the body to maintain its alignment over time.

- **The Adjustment Process**: NUCCA adjustments are performed without any popping, cracking, or sudden movements. Instead, the practitioner uses gentle pressure to realign the Atlas, based on precise measurements taken from X-rays. The adjustment is so gentle that many patients are surprised by how little they feel during the procedure—yet the results can be life-changing.

- **Patient Success Stories**: NUCCA has helped thousands of people overcome chronic health issues related to Atlas misalignment. From severe migraines and vertigo to scoliosis and TMJ disorders, patients have reported significant improvements in their symptoms after just a few NUCCA adjustments. These success stories highlight the power of subtle, precise adjustments in restoring health and well-being.

AtlasPROfilax®: A Unique Approach to Atlas Realignment

"One adjustment, one life-changing moment."

The **AtlasPROfilax® method**, developed by Swiss medical researcher René-Claudius Schümperli in the 1990s, offers a unique approach to Atlas correction. For instance, **Yves Humbert**, a specialist in this method, has received formal training in it. Unlike AO and NUCCA, which often involve multiple sessions,

AtlasPROfilax® is designed to realign the Atlas in just one session.

This method has gained popularity in Europe and other parts of the world for its simplicity and effectiveness.

- **Origins of AtlasPROfilax®**: Schümperli developed the AtlasPROfilax® method after suffering from severe spinal issues himself. After years of research, he discovered that a single, precise adjustment to the Atlas could provide lasting relief from a wide range of symptoms. The method is based on the idea that once the Atlas is properly aligned, the body can naturally maintain this alignment, reducing the need for ongoing adjustments.

- **How It Works**: The *AtlasPROfilax®* adjustment is performed using a specialized device that applies targeted pressure to the muscles surrounding the Atlas. This pressure helps to gently guide the Atlas back into its correct position. The procedure is quick, usually lasting only a few minutes, and does not involve any forceful manipulation of the spine.

- **Long-Term Results**: One of the key benefits of *AtlasPROfilax®* is its potential for long-term results. Many patients report significant improvements in their symptoms after just one session, with no need for further adjustments. This makes it an attractive option for those looking for a one-time solution to their Atlas-related health issues.

- **Global Reach**: AtlasPROfilax® has practitioners around the world, and its popularity continues to grow as more people experience its benefits. From Europe to Asia to the Americas, this method has helped countless individuals regain their health and quality of life by addressing Atlas misalignment in a simple, effective way.

Other Holistic Approaches to Atlas Health

"The whole is greater than the sum of its parts." — *Aristotle*

While AO, NUCCA, and **AtlasPROfilax®** are among the most well-known methods for Atlas correction, there are other **holistic** approaches that can complement these techniques and support overall spinal health. These methods often focus on maintaining the alignment of the Atlas through lifestyle changes, exercises, and complementary therapies.

- **Craniosacral Therapy**: This gentle, hands-on approach to treatment involves manipulating the cranial bones, including the Atlas, to relieve tension and improve the flow of cerebrospinal fluid. Craniosacral therapy can be particularly beneficial for patients with chronic pain, headaches, or stress-related disorders, as it helps to restore balance and promote relaxation.

- **Yoga and Stretching**: Yoga and targeted stretching exercises can help maintain the alignment of the Atlas by strengthening the muscles that support the neck and improving posture.

Specific poses, such as the Cat-Cow and Child's Pose, are designed to elongate the spine and encourage proper alignment.

- **Postural Training**: Postural training programs, such as the Alexander Technique or the Egoscue Method, can help individuals become more aware of their posture and movement patterns, reducing the risk of Atlas misalignment. By learning how to move and sit in ways that support spinal health, patients can prevent the recurrence of misalignment.

- **Massage Therapy**: Regular massage therapy can help to relieve muscle tension and support Atlas alignment. Techniques such as deep tissue massage and myofascial release target the muscles surrounding the Atlas, helping to keep them relaxed and preventing tightness that can lead to misalignment.

Choosing the Right Approach for You

"The journey to wellness is personal—choose the path that resonates with you."

With so many options available, it's important to choose the approach to Atlas correction that best suits your needs and preferences. Here are some considerations to help you make an informed decision:

- **Severity of Symptoms**: If you're experiencing severe or debilitating symptoms, a more precise approach like AO or NUCCA may be the best option. These methods are designed to provide targeted relief and can be tailored to address specific misalignments, especially in the USA.

- **Personal Preferences**: Some people prefer a more hands-on approach, while others may feel more comfortable with a gentle, non-invasive method. Consider your comfort level with different techniques and choose a practitioner who aligns with your preferences such as **Yves Humbert** in Europe.

- **Lifestyle and Maintenance**: If you're looking for a one-time solution, **AtlasPROfilax®** might be the right choice.

- However, if you're committed to ongoing maintenance and lifestyle changes, a method like NUCCA, combined with complementary therapies, could provide long-term benefits.

- **Availability of Practitioners**: Depending on where you live, certain methods may be more accessible than others. Research local practitioners and consider traveling if necessary to receive the care that best meets your needs. (See our list)

Conclusion: The Path to Realignment

Atlas misalignment may be a hidden cause of many chronic health issues, but it doesn't have to remain hidden forever. With the right approach, you can correct your alignment, restore balance to your body, and reclaim your health. Whether through the precision of Atlas Orthogonal, the gentle touch of NUCCA, or the simplicity of **AtlasPROfilax®,** there's a path to realignment that's right for you.

In the next chapter, we'll explore self-regulation and regeneration techniques that you can use at home to support your Atlas alignment and enhance your overall well-being. These tools, combined with professional care, will empower you to take control of your health and enjoy a life free from the limitations of Atlas misalignment.

Chapter 4: Self-Regulation and Regeneration: How to Heal Yourself

"Healing is a matter of time, but it is sometimes also a matter of opportunity." — *Hippocrates*

The process of healing is multifaceted, involving not just the correction of physical misalignments but also the ongoing care and maintenance of the body. Once you've taken the crucial step of addressing your Atlas misalignment with the help of a professional, the journey doesn't end there. To sustain the benefits and prevent future issues, it's essential to incorporate self-regulation and regeneration techniques into your daily life.

The Importance of Posture: Aligning Your Life

"Stand up straight and realize who you are, that you tower over your circumstances." — *Maya Angelou*

One of the simplest yet most effective ways to maintain Atlas alignment is through **proper posture**. How you sit, stand, and move throughout the day has a significant impact on your spinal health. Poor posture can strain the muscles and ligaments that support your Atlas, potentially leading to misalignment. Let's explore some key strategies for maintaining good posture and supporting your Atlas.

- **Sitting Posture**: Whether you're working at a desk, watching TV, or eating a meal, how you sit matters. Ensure that your chair provides adequate support for your lower back, and **keep your feet flat on the floor with your knees at a 90-degree angle**. Your head should be aligned with your spine, and your shoulders relaxed. Consider using a lumbar roll or ergonomic chair to maintain the natural curve of your lower spine, which in turn supports your cervical spine and Atlas.

- **Standing Posture**: When standing, distribute your weight evenly between both feet. Avoid slouching or leaning to one side, as this can cause uneven pressure on your spine and lead to misalignment. Keep your head level, your shoulders back, and your abdominal muscles engaged. **<u>Imagine a string pulling you up from the top of your head</u>**—this mental image can help you maintain a tall, aligned posture.

- **Ergonomic Workspaces**: For those who spend long hours at a desk, an ergonomic workspace is essential. Position your computer screen at eye level to avoid tilting your head forward. Use a chair that supports your lumbar spine, and ensure that your keyboard and mouse are within easy reach to prevent straining your shoulders and neck. It is also recommended to take breaks every 90 minutes, get up, and go for a walk (and not just for a coffee with your colleagues!)

Movement and Exercise beyond 90 minutes break : Strengthening Your Support System

"Movement is a medicine for creating change in a person's physical, emotional, and mental states." — *Carol Welch*

Regular exercise is vital for maintaining the alignment of your Atlas and supporting overall spinal health. By strengthening the muscles that support your neck and spine, you can reduce the risk of future misalignment and improve your body's ability to heal itself. Here are some exercises that are particularly beneficial for maintaining Atlas alignment.

- **Neck Stretches**: Gentle neck stretches can help maintain flexibility and prevent stiffness in the muscles surrounding the Atlas. Try the following exercises:
    - **Chin Tucks**: Sit or stand with your back straight and gently tuck your chin towards your chest, keeping your shoulders relaxed. Hold for a few seconds, then return to the starting position. Repeat 10 times.
    - **Side-to-Side Head Turns**: Slowly turn your head to the left as far as is comfortable, then return to the center. Repeat on the right side. Perform 10 repetitions on each side.
    - **Neck Tilts**: Tilt your head towards your shoulder, bringing your ear as close as possible without lifting your shoulder. Hold for a few seconds, then return to the center and repeat on the other side. Do 10 repetitions on each side.
- **Core Strengthening**: A strong core supports the spine and helps maintain proper alignment. Incorporate exercises like planks, bridges, and abdominal crunches into your routine to build core strength. These exercises help stabilize your pelvis and lower back, reducing the strain on your neck and upper spine.

- **Yoga and Pilates**: Both yoga and Pilates focus on core strength, flexibility, and body awareness—all of which are crucial for maintaining Atlas alignment. Specific yoga poses, such as the Cat-Cow, Downward Dog, and Child's Pose, help elongate the spine and improve posture. Pilates exercises emphasize controlled movements and core engagement, which support spinal stability.

- **Aerobic Exercise**: Regular aerobic exercise, such as walking, swimming, or cycling, promotes overall health and well-being. It improves circulation, helps maintain a healthy weight, and reduces stress—factors that all contribute to spinal health and prevent Atlas misalignment.

Breathing and Relaxation Techniques: Calming the Nervous System

"Breath is the bridge which connects life to consciousness, which unites your body to your thoughts." — *Thích Nhất Hạnh*

The connection between the breath and the nervous system is profound. Deep, mindful breathing can help calm the nervous system, reduce tension in the muscles surrounding the Atlas, and promote overall relaxation. Here are some breathing and relaxation techniques that can support your Atlas health.

- **Diaphragmatic Breathing**: Also known as belly breathing, diaphragmatic breathing engages the diaphragm and allows for deeper, more efficient breaths. This type of breathing can reduce tension in the neck and shoulders, areas often affected by Atlas misalignment.

- ○ **How to Practice**: Sit or lie down in a comfortable position. Place one hand on your chest and the other on your abdomen. Breathe in slowly through your nose, allowing your abdomen to rise while keeping your chest still. Exhale slowly through your mouth, letting your abdomen fall. Repeat for 5–10 minutes, focusing on the rise and fall of your abdomen.
- **Progressive Muscle Relaxation (PMR)**: PMR is a technique that involves tensing and then relaxing different muscle groups in the body. This method can help release tension in the muscles surrounding the Atlas and promote overall relaxation.
  - ○ **How to Practice**: Starting with your toes, tense the muscles in that area for 5 seconds, then slowly release. Move up through your body, tensing and relaxing each muscle group, including your legs, abdomen, arms, and neck. Pay special attention to the muscles around your neck and shoulders, which often hold tension related to Atlas misalignment.
- **Mindful Meditation**: Meditation can help reduce stress, which is a common contributor to muscle tension and spinal misalignment. Regular meditation practice can promote a sense of calm and well-being, supporting your body's ability to maintain Atlas alignment.
  - ○ **How to Practice**: Find a quiet space and sit comfortably. Close your eyes and focus on your breath, noticing the sensation of the air entering and leaving your nostrils (5 times deeply) . If your mind wanders, gently bring your attention back to your breath. Start with 5 minutes a day (5 breathing minimum) and gradually increase the duration (to 15 minutes) as you become more comfortable with the practice.

Nutritional Support: Feeding Your Spine

"Let food be thy medicine and medicine be thy food." — *Hippocrates*

Nutrition plays a crucial role in maintaining the health of your spine and supporting the healing process after Atlas correction. A balanced diet rich in essential nutrients can help reduce inflammation, support muscle and bone health, and promote overall wellness.

- **Anti-Inflammatory Foods**: Chronic inflammation can contribute to pain and stiffness in the muscles and joints, making it harder to maintain Atlas alignment. Incorporate anti-inflammatory foods into your diet, such as:
    - **Fatty Fish**: Salmon, mackerel, and sardines are rich in Omega-3 fatty acids, which have powerful anti-inflammatory effects.
    - **Leafy Greens**: Spinach, kale, and Swiss chard are packed with antioxidants that help combat inflammation.
    - **Berries**: **<u>Blueberries</u>**, strawberries, and blackberries contain flavonoids that reduce inflammation and support immune health.
    - **Nuts and Seeds**: Almonds, walnuts, and flaxseeds are good sources of healthy fats and antioxidants.
- **Calcium and Vitamin D**: These nutrients are essential for maintaining strong bones and preventing osteoporosis, which can affect spinal health. Ensure you're getting enough calcium from dairy products, leafy greens, and fortified foods, and vitamin D from sunlight exposure, fatty fish, and supplements if needed.

- **Magnesium**: Magnesium is important for muscle relaxation and nerve function. Foods rich in magnesium include dark chocolate, avocados, nuts, seeds, and whole grains. Adequate magnesium intake can help prevent muscle cramps and tension, which are often associated with Atlas misalignment.

- **Hydration**: Staying well-hydrated is crucial for maintaining the health of your spinal discs, which act as cushions between your vertebrae. Aim to drink at least eight glasses of water a day, and more if you're active or live in a hot climate.

Tools and Aids: Supporting Your Atlas at Home

"The right tools make all the difference."

In addition to lifestyle changes, there are various tools and aids that can help you maintain Atlas alignment and support your spinal health. These products are designed to reduce strain on your neck and spine, promote proper posture, and enhance your overall comfort.

- **Ergonomic Pillows**: A good pillow can make a significant difference in maintaining Atlas alignment while you sleep. Look for a pillow that supports the natural curve of your neck and keeps your head in a neutral position. Memory foam or cervical pillows are popular choices for those with neck issues.

- **Posture Correctors**: Posture correctors are wearable devices that help you maintain proper alignment throughout the day. They gently pull your shoulders back and align your spine, reducing the risk of slouching or poor posture that could affect your Atlas.

- **Foam Rollers**: Foam rollers can be used to release tension in the muscles surrounding the Atlas and spine. Regular foam rolling can help improve flexibility, reduce muscle tightness, and support overall spinal health. Focus on rolling out the upper back, shoulders, and neck to relieve tension.

- **Neck Braces**: In some cases, a neck brace may be recommended to support the cervical spine and prevent further misalignment. Neck braces can be used temporarily after an Atlas adjustment to help maintain alignment, especially if you're recovering from an injury or surgery.

Holistic Practices: Integrating Body, Mind, and Spirit

"True healing involves treating the whole person, NOT just the symptoms."

To achieve lasting health and maintain Atlas alignment, it's important to take a holistic approach that considers the connection between body, mind, and spirit. Integrating these practices into your daily routine can help you cultivate a sense of balance and well-being that supports your physical health.

- **Mind-Body Therapies**: Mind-body therapies, such as tai chi, qigong, and acupuncture, can help promote relaxation, reduce stress, and support spinal health. These practices emphasize the flow of energy (chi) throughout the body and can be particularly beneficial for those dealing with chronic pain or tension related to Atlas misalignment.

- **Spiritual Practices**: For many, spiritual practices such as prayer, meditation, or mindfulness play a key role in overall well-being. These practices can help you connect with a deeper sense of purpose and inner peace, which can, in turn, support your physical health. Consider incorporating daily meditation, journaling, or time spent in nature as part of your self-care routine.

- **Visualization and Affirmations**: Visualization techniques and positive affirmations can be powerful tools for promoting healing and maintaining alignment. Visualize your spine and Atlas in perfect alignment, and repeat affirmations such as, "I am strong, balanced, and aligned," to reinforce a positive mindset.

Conclusion: Empowering Your Healing Journey

"The greatest medicine of all is teaching people how not to need it." — *Hippocrates*

Healing is not a one-time event but a continuous journey. By integrating self-regulation and regeneration techniques into your daily life, you can support your Atlas alignment, enhance your overall well-being, and prevent future health issues. Remember, the key to lasting health lies in maintaining balance—physically, mentally, and emotionally.

As you continue your healing journey, take pride in the steps you're taking to care for your body and mind. By making these practices a regular part of your life, you're not only supporting your Atlas alignment but also empowering yourself to live a healthier, happier life. But, where to go ?

References:

1. *Haines, D. E. (2012). Neuroanatomy: An Atlas of Structures, Sections, and Systems (8th ed.). Wolters Kluwer Health/Lippincott Williams & Wilkins.*

2. *Gordon, R., & Bloxham, S. (2016). A Systematic Review of the Effects of Exercise and Physical Activity on Non-Specific Chronic Low Back Pain. Healthcare, 4(2), 22. Retrieved from ncbi.nlm.nih.gov*

3. *Lee, D. Y., & Kim, J. (2019). Effects of Diaphragmatic Breathing on the Stabilization of the Cervical Spine. Journal of Physical Therapy Science, 31(5), 384-388. Retrieved from jstage.jst.go.jp*

4. *Leach, R. A. (2004). The Chiropractic Theories: A Textbook of Scientific Research (4th ed.). Lippincott Williams & Wilkins.*

5. *Kaptchuk, T. J. (2002). Acupuncture: Theory, Efficacy, and Practice. Annals of Internal Medicine, 136(5), 374-383. Retrieved from acpjournals.org*

Chapter 5: Atlas Healing: A Global Phenomenon

"Healing is not just a science, it's an art. It doesn't come from the intellect, it comes from the heart." — *Aziz Shaman*

The understanding and practice of Atlas correction have transcended borders, becoming a global movement in the pursuit of holistic health. As awareness of the Atlas bone's critical role in well-being grows, more people across the world are turning to specialized practitioners to help them realign their lives—literally and figuratively. In this chapter, we'll introduce you to some of the leading Atlas practitioners around the globe, each of whom has made a significant impact on the field. We'll also explore the diverse methods they use, the philosophies that guide them, and the life-changing stories of their patients.

United States: Dr. Jeff McGuckin

"**Precision in healing requires both skill and heart.**"

Dr. Jeff McGuckin is a renowned Atlas Orthogonal chiropractor based in Atlanta, Georgia. His approach to Atlas correction is characterized by meticulous attention to detail and a deep commitment to his patients' overall well-being. Trained directly under **Dr. Roy Sweat**, the founder of the Atlas Orthogonal technique, **Dr. McGuckin** has spent decades refining his practice to achieve the highest levels of precision and care.

- **Atlas Orthogonal Technique**: **Dr. McGuckin** specializes in the Atlas Orthogonal technique, which uses a precise instrument to adjust the Atlas without any manual manipulation. This technique is based on advanced imaging and mathematical calculations to ensure that the adjustment is tailored specifically to the patient's needs. The result is a gentle, yet effective correction that can alleviate a wide range of symptoms, from chronic pain to neurological disorders.

- **Patient Success Stories**: Many of **Dr. McGuckin's** patients have experienced dramatic improvements in their health after undergoing Atlas Orthogonal treatment. One such patient, Lisa, suffered from debilitating migraines for years. After just a few sessions with **Dr. McGuckin,** her migraines were significantly reduced, and she was able to return to a normal life without the need for medication.

- **Philosophy of Care**: **Dr. McGuckin** believes that healing goes beyond just correcting physical misalignments. He emphasizes the importance of a holistic approach, integrating lifestyle changes, nutrition, and stress management into his treatment plans. His goal is to empower his patients to take control of their health and achieve long-term well-being.

Canada: Dr. Dennis Poole

"True health is about balance—both in the body and in life."

In Toronto, Canada, Dr. Dennis Poole has become a leading figure in the field of upper cervical chiropractic care. His clinic, known for its state-of-the-art facilities and compassionate care, attracts patients from across the country who are seeking relief from chronic conditions.

- **Upper Cervical Chiropractic**: Dr. Poole's approach focuses on the upper cervical spine, particularly the Atlas and axis vertebrae. Using advanced imaging techniques such as cone-beam CT scans, Dr. Poole can precisely diagnose and correct misalignments that are often missed by traditional chiropractic methods. His gentle adjustments are designed to restore balance to the nervous system, allowing the body to heal itself naturally.

- **Innovative Techniques**: Dr. Poole integrates cutting-edge technology with time-tested chiropractic principles. He is known for his use of digital motion X-rays, which allow him to see how the vertebrae move in real-time, providing a more accurate diagnosis and treatment plan. This innovation has led to remarkable results, particularly for patients with complex or long-standing issues.

- **Patient Testimonials**: One of Dr. Poole's patients, Mark, had been suffering from severe vertigo for years, which had severely limited his ability to work and enjoy life. After a thorough assessment and a series of precise adjustments, Mark's vertigo dramatically improved, and he was able to resume his normal activities. Mark credits Dr. Poole's expertise and care with giving him his life back.

Switzerland: Yves Humbert

"Healing is about restoring harmony within the body, and that begins with the Atlas." *Yves Humbert, August 2024, Sion (CH)*

Yves Humbert is a leading figure in the field of Atlas correction in Europe. Based in *Sion, Switzerland*, Yves has been practicing for over two decades, utilizing a specialized machine, along with a portable table passed down from his teacher, to carry out precise Atlas adjustments. His work has brought life-changing results to numerous individuals who had previously given up hope of finding relief, such as *Angela,* who was transformed by his treatment as detailed in earlier case studies.

- **Patient Transformations**: Yves has helped countless patients who were suffering from chronic pain, migraines, and neurological disorders in Switzerland. One such patient, Sophie, had been experiencing severe neck pain and numbness in her arms for years. After her treatment with Yves, she not only found relief from her symptoms but also experienced a newfound sense of balance and well-being.

- **Philosophy and Approach**: Yves believes that healing is a holistic process that involves not just the body, but also the mind and spirit. His approach integrates physical adjustments with guidance on lifestyle changes, including diet, exercise, and stress management. Yves' practice is a testament to the power of combining traditional wisdom with modern technology.

Australia: Dr. Luke Korthals

"Alignment is the foundation of health, and it starts with the Atlas."

Dr. Luke Korthals is a leading Atlas chiropractor in Melbourne, Australia. He specializes in the **AtlasPROfilax®** method, which offers a unique approach to Atlas correction. His work has garnered a loyal following, particularly among those who have tried multiple other treatments without success.

- **AtlasPROfilax® Method**: The **AtlasPROfilax®** method, developed by René-Claudius Schümperli, is a one-time adjustment technique that aims to realign the Atlas in a single session. **Dr. Korthals** is one of the few practitioners in Australia trained in this method. The procedure involves applying targeted pressure to the muscles surrounding the Atlas, allowing it to return to its correct position naturally.

- **Patient Experiences**: Many of **Dr. Korthals'** patients have experienced life-changing results after just one session. For example, Sarah, a long-time sufferer of chronic back pain and migraines, found immediate relief after her **AtlasPROfilax®** treatment. She reported not only a reduction in pain but also an overall improvement in her posture and energy levels.

- **Holistic Health Focus**: **Dr. Korthals** emphasizes the importance of maintaining the benefits of the **AtlasPROfilax®** adjustment through a healthy lifestyle. He provides his patients with guidance on nutrition, exercise, and mindfulness practices that support long-term health and prevent future misalignments.

United Kingdom: Dr. Michael Burcon

"The Atlas is the key to unlocking the body's natural healing potential."

In the UK, Dr. Michael Burcon is a respected upper cervical chiropractor with a practice in London. His work focuses on the **NUCCA** (*National Upper Cervical Chiropractic Association*) method, which offers a gentle, non-invasive approach to Atlas correction.

- **NUCCA Technique**: The NUCCA method is based on precise measurements and gentle adjustments designed to restore balance to the spine and nervous system. *Dr. Burcon*'s approach is particularly effective for patients with conditions like Meniere's disease, vertigo, and chronic migraines. By correcting the alignment of the Atlas, he helps his patients achieve relief from symptoms that have often been resistant to other forms of treatment.

- **Scientific Approach**: *Dr. Burcon* is known for his rigorous, evidence-based approach to chiropractic care. He often collaborates with researchers and other healthcare professionals to advance the understanding of upper cervical care and its impact on overall health. His commitment to science and patient care has made him a trusted name in the field.

- **Patient Stories**: One of *Dr. Burcon*'s notable successes involved a patient named Emily, who had been diagnosed with Meniere's disease and was struggling with severe dizziness and hearing loss. After a series of *NUCCA* adjustments, Emily's symptoms improved significantly, and she regained much of her quality of life. Her story is one of many that highlight the effectiveness of the *NUCCA* method in treating complex conditions.

India: Dr. Deepak Kumar

"The Atlas is where true healing begins."

Dr. Deepak Kumar, based in Mumbai, India, is one of the few practitioners in the country specializing in Atlas orthogonal chiropractic care. His approach combines modern chiropractic techniques with the rich traditions of Indian holistic medicine, offering a unique blend of Eastern and Western healing.

- **Atlas Orthogonal in India**: Dr. Kumar's practice focuses on the **Atlas Orthogonal technique,** which is relatively new to India but has quickly gained recognition for its effectiveness. By using a precise, instrument-based adjustment, Dr. Kumar is able to correct misalignments without the need for manual manipulation. This technique is particularly appealing to patients who are hesitant about traditional chiropractic methods.

- **Integration with Ayurveda**: Dr. Kumar integrates principles of Ayurveda, India's ancient system of medicine, into his practice. He believes that the key to long-term health lies in balancing the body's doshas (vital energies) and that Atlas alignment plays a crucial role in this balance. His treatment plans often include dietary recommendations, herbal supplements, and yoga practices that support the body's natural healing processes.

- **Success Stories**: One of Dr. Kumar's patients, Priya, had been suffering from chronic fatigue and fibromyalgia. Traditional treatments had provided little relief, but after undergoing Atlas orthogonal adjustments combined with Ayurvedic therapies, Priya experienced a significant reduction in her symptoms. She was able to regain her energy and return to her daily activities with renewed vigor.

Germany: Dr. Thomas Rau

"Balance in the body begins with the balance of the spine."

Dr. Thomas Rau, located in *Stuttgart, Germany*, is a leading expert in Atlas chiropractic care, particularly known for his work with athletes and individuals with complex health issues. His clinic is a hub for those seeking advanced chiropractic care in Europe.

- **Specialized Care for Athletes**: *Dr. Rau* has developed a reputation for his work with professional athletes who require precise and effective treatments to maintain peak performance. His approach to Atlas correction is tailored to the specific needs of athletes, helping them recover from injuries, prevent future issues, and optimize their physical capabilities.

- **Holistic Health Programs**: *Dr. Rau's* clinic offers comprehensive health programs that combine Atlas chiropractic care with other modalities, such as physical therapy, nutritional counseling, and functional medicine. This integrative approach ensures that patients receive well-rounded care that addresses all aspects of their health.

- **Patient Impact**: One of *Dr. Rau's* notable patients, a professional football player, had been dealing with chronic neck pain that was affecting his performance on the field. After undergoing a series of Atlas adjustments and participating in a personalized health program, he experienced significant improvements in his pain levels, mobility, and overall performance. This success story is just one example of how Dr. Rau's expertise in Atlas care can make a difference for individuals with demanding physical requirements.

Spain: Dr. Eduardo López

"The body has the capacity to heal itself, but it needs the right alignment to do so."

Dr. Eduardo López, a respected Atlas specialist in Madrid, Spain, has helped many patients find relief from chronic health issues through his expertise in upper cervical care. His practice is known for its focus on personalized care and patient education.

- **Atlas Orthogonal Expertise**: Dr. López's clinic is one of the few in Spain offering the Atlas Orthogonal technique. He is dedicated to using the most precise and gentle methods available to correct Atlas misalignments. His patients often remark on the thoroughness of his approach and the time he takes to ensure that each adjustment is tailored to their specific needs.

- **Education and Empowerment**: Dr. López believes that patient education is a key component of effective treatment. He takes the time to explain the importance of Atlas alignment and how it affects overall health. By empowering his patients with knowledge, he helps them take an active role in their healing journey.

- **Patient Experiences**: One of Dr. López's patients, Javier, had been suffering from chronic neck pain and headaches for years. After undergoing Atlas orthogonal adjustments, Javier noticed a significant reduction in his symptoms. He also appreciated the education and support he received from Dr. López, which helped him make lifestyle changes that supported his long-term health.

Italy: Dr. Alessandro Bolognesi

"Health is not just the absence of disease, but the presence of alignment."

In Rome, Italy, ***Dr. Alessandro Bolognesi*** has built a reputation as one of the country's leading Atlas orthogonal chiropractors. His clinic is a center of excellence for patients suffering from severe spinal issues, including scoliosis and degenerative disc disease.

- **Atlas Orthogonal in Italy**: *Dr. Bolognesi's* practice is distinguished by its focus on precision and patient-centered care. He uses the Atlas Orthogonal technique to address misalignments that are often at the root of chronic spinal conditions. His approach is known for its effectiveness in reducing pain and improving spinal function.

- **Advanced Diagnostic Tools**: *Dr. Bolognesi's* clinic is equipped with the latest diagnostic tools, including digital X-rays and motion analysis systems. These technologies allow him to assess the full extent of a patient's spinal issues and develop a comprehensive treatment plan that addresses both the symptoms and the underlying causes.

- **Patient Success Stories**: *Dr. Bolognesi's* work has transformed the lives of many patients, including Lucia, who had been living with severe scoliosis and chronic back pain. After undergoing a series of Atlas orthogonal adjustments and participating in a rehabilitation program, Lucia experienced significant improvements in her pain levels and mobility. She was able to return to activities she had previously thought impossible, thanks to Dr. Bolognesi's care.

Global Impact: The Growing Awareness of Atlas Health

"The Atlas is the bridge between the body and the world."

The work of these practitioners across different continents highlights the universal importance of the Atlas bone in maintaining overall health. Their dedication and diverse approaches reflect a growing global awareness of the crucial role the Atlas plays in our well-being. As more people discover the benefits of Atlas correction, the field continues to expand, bringing new innovations and greater understanding to this vital area of healthcare.

The Future of Atlas Healing

"Healing is an ever-evolving art, informed by the past and guided by the future."

As awareness of Atlas health continues to grow, so too does the potential for new developments and innovations in the field. Researchers and practitioners are constantly exploring new techniques, technologies, and approaches to improve the effectiveness of Atlas correction and make it more accessible to people around the world.

- **Wearable Technology**: The future of Atlas care may include wearable devices that monitor spinal alignment and provide feedback to help patients maintain proper posture throughout the day. These devices could be particularly useful for preventing misalignments before they cause symptoms.

- **Telemedicine**: With the rise of telemedicine, Atlas practitioners are finding new ways to reach and treat patients remotely. This technology allows for virtual consultations, follow-ups, and even guided self-assessment, making Atlas care more accessible to those in remote areas or with limited mobility.

- **Continued Research**: Ongoing research into the effects of Atlas alignment on various health conditions is helping to build a stronger evidence base for its benefits. As more studies are conducted, we can expect to see a greater integration of Atlas care into mainstream healthcare practices.

Conclusion: The Global Movement Toward Atlas Health

"Health is a journey that we take together, across borders and through time."

The practice of Atlas correction has truly become a global phenomenon, with practitioners from diverse backgrounds and regions contributing to the advancement of this field. Whether in the United States, Canada, Switzerland, Australia, the United Kingdom, India, Germany, Spain, or Italy, the common thread that unites these practitioners is their commitment to helping people achieve optimal health through the power of Atlas alignment.

As we've seen, the impact of Atlas correction can be profound, transforming lives and restoring balance to the body. The stories and experiences shared in this chapter are just a few examples of how this powerful approach to healing is making a difference around the world.

We will explore the causes of Atlas joint instability, the consequences of leaving it untreated, and the solutions available to stabilize the Atlas and prevent future misalignments. We'll dive deeper into the biomechanics of the Atlas and how you can take proactive steps to support your spinal health.

References:

1. *Sweat, R. W. (2007). Atlas Orthogonal Chiropractic: Advanced Orthogonal Procedures (2nd ed.). Chiropractic Health Press.*

2. *Eriksen, K., & Rochester, R. (2011). Upper Cervical Subluxation Complex: A Review of the Chiropractic and Medical Literature. Lippincott Williams & Wilkins.*

3. *Senzon, S. A. (2002). Chiropractic Perspectives: The Evolution of a Profession. Foundation for Vertebral Subluxation.*

4. *Schümperli, R. C. (1996). AtlasPROfilax®: The Schümperli Method. Swiss Academy of Natural Medicine.*

5. *Rau, T. (2018). The Bioregulatory Medicine Approach: Toward Complete Health and Wellness. Bioregulatory Medicine Press.*

6. *Y.Humbert (2024) . Atlas the Revolution on the Way.*

Chapter 6: Atlas Joint Instability (Scientific chapter)
Causes, Consequences, and Solutions

**"A chain is only as strong as its weakest link.
In the body, the Atlas is that link."**

The Atlas vertebra, as the cornerstone of the cervical spine, plays a crucial role in maintaining the stability and alignment of the entire spinal column. However, like any cornerstone, if the Atlas becomes unstable, the repercussions can be felt throughout the body. In this chapter, we will explore the causes of Atlas joint instability, the consequences of leaving it untreated, and the various solutions available to restore and maintain stability.

What is Atlas Joint Instability?

"Atlas joint instability is like a faulty foundation. Without correction, the structure above it will eventually crumble."

Atlas joint instability refers to a condition where the Atlas vertebra (**C1**) does not maintain its proper alignment or position relative to the axis (**C2**) and the base of the skull. This instability can result from various factors, including trauma, degenerative changes, and congenital anomalies. When the Atlas is unstable, it can lead to excessive movement (hypermobility) or improper alignment, which in turn can cause a range of symptoms and health issues.

- **Hypermobility vs. Hypomobility**: Hypermobility occurs when the Atlas moves more than it should, leading to excessive strain on the surrounding ligaments and muscles. Hypomobility, on the other hand, is when the Atlas is restricted in its movement, which can also lead to dysfunction and compensatory issues in the surrounding structures. Both conditions can contribute to instability, albeit in different ways.

- **Common Causes of Instability**: Atlas joint instability can be caused by various factors, including:
    - **Trauma**: Whiplash injuries from car accidents, falls, or sports injuries can damage the ligaments and muscles that support the Atlas, leading to instability.
    - **Degenerative Changes**: Age-related wear and tear, such as arthritis, can weaken the structures that hold the Atlas in place, making it more prone to instability.
    - **Congenital Anomalies**: Some people are born with anatomical differences that predispose them to Atlas instability, such as a malformed dens (odontoid process) or an underdeveloped Atlas.
    - **Chronic Poor Posture**: Long-term poor posture, such as forward head posture or slouching, can strain the neck muscles and ligaments, leading to instability over time.

The Consequences of Atlas Joint Instability

"When the Atlas is unstable, the body compensates—but at a cost."

The consequences of leaving Atlas joint instability untreated can be far-reaching. Because the Atlas is the top vertebra of the spine and supports the skull, any instability here can have a cascading effect on the rest of the body.

- **Musculoskeletal Imbalance**: When the Atlas is unstable, the body often compensates by altering the posture and mechanics of the entire spine. This can lead to muscle imbalances, joint strain, and misalignments throughout the body. Over time, these compensations can contribute to chronic pain, stiffness, and mobility issues.

- **Neurological Symptoms**: The Atlas is located at the junction where the spinal cord exits the brainstem, making it a critical area for nervous system function. Instability in the Atlas can lead to compression or irritation of the spinal cord and surrounding nerves, resulting in symptoms such as headaches, dizziness, vertigo, and even sensory or motor disturbances in the limbs.

- **Vascular Impairment**: The vertebral arteries pass through the transverse foramina of the cervical vertebrae, including the Atlas. If the Atlas is unstable, it can impinge on these arteries, reducing blood flow to the brain. This can lead to symptoms such as blurred vision, fainting, and cognitive impairments like brain fog.

- **Chronic Pain and Fatigue**: The constant strain on the neck muscles and ligaments due to Atlas instability can lead to

chronic pain conditions such as **cervicalgia (neck pain)** and cervicogenic headaches.

- Diagnosing Atlas Joint Instability

"The first step to fixing a problem is understanding it."

Diagnosing Atlas joint instability can be challenging, as the symptoms often overlap with other conditions, and the instability itself may not be immediately apparent. However, with the right tools and techniques, practitioners can accurately identify Atlas instability and develop an effective treatment plan.

- **Imaging Techniques**: Advanced imaging techniques, such as dynamic X-rays, MRI, and CT scans, are often used to assess Atlas stability. Dynamic imaging (taken while the neck is in motion) is particularly useful for identifying hypermobility or other abnormal movements of the Atlas that may not be visible in static images.

- **Neurological Examination**: A thorough neurological examination can help identify any sensory or motor deficits that may be related to Atlas instability. This examination may include tests for reflexes, muscle strength, coordination, and balance, all of which can be affected by issues in the upper cervical spine.

- **Posture and Movement Analysis**: Postural assessments and gait analysis can provide valuable insights into how Atlas instability is affecting the body's overall mechanics. Practitioners may use these assessments to identify compensatory patterns and areas of muscle tension that indicate instability.

- **Patient History and Symptom Review**: A detailed patient history, including any past injuries, chronic symptoms, and lifestyle factors, is crucial for diagnosing Atlas instability. Understanding the patient's experience and how their symptoms have developed over time can help guide the diagnostic process and treatment plan.

Solutions for Atlas Joint Instability

"Stability is the foundation of health."

Once Atlas instability has been diagnosed, the next step is to stabilize the joint and restore proper alignment. A combination of targeted treatments and lifestyle changes can help achieve this goal, allowing the body to heal and function optimally.

- **Chiropractic Care**: Chiropractic adjustments, particularly those focused on the upper cervical spine, can be highly effective in stabilizing the Atlas. Techniques like Atlas Orthogonal, NUCCA, and Blair Upper Cervical are specifically designed to address Atlas misalignment and instability with precise, gentle adjustments. Regular chiropractic care can help maintain Atlas alignment and prevent future instability.

- **Physical Therapy**: Physical therapy plays a key role in strengthening the muscles that support the neck and improving overall stability. A physical therapist may prescribe exercises to strengthen the deep neck flexors, which are crucial for maintaining proper head and neck alignment. They may also work on improving posture and flexibility to reduce strain on the Atlas and surrounding structures.

- **Prolotherapy and PRP Injections**: For patients with significant ligament damage or chronic instability, regenerative therapies like prolotherapy or platelet-rich plasma (PRP) injections may be recommended. These treatments involve injecting natural substances into the affected ligaments to promote healing and strengthen the tissues, thereby enhancing joint stability.

- **Lifestyle Modifications**: Making changes to daily habits can significantly impact Atlas stability. This may include ergonomic adjustments to your workspace, improving your sleep posture, and incorporating regular exercise and stretching routines that support spinal health. Avoiding activities that place excessive strain on the neck, such as heavy lifting or prolonged use of electronic devices, can also help maintain stability.

- **Bracing and Supportive Devices**: In some cases, a cervical collar or neck brace may be used temporarily to provide additional support and allow the ligaments and muscles to heal. These devices are typically used in conjunction with other treatments and are not intended for long-term use, as they can lead to muscle weakening if relied upon for too long.

Preventing Future Instability

"An ounce of prevention is worth a pound of cure." —
Benjamin Franklin

Preventing Atlas joint instability from recurring is just as important as treating it. By taking proactive steps to protect your spine and maintain good posture, you can reduce the risk of future instability and ensure that your body remains balanced and healthy.

- **Ergonomic Practices**: Maintaining an ergonomic workspace and using supportive furniture can go a long way in preventing neck strain and maintaining Atlas stability. Ensure that your computer screen is at eye level, your chair supports your lower back, and you take regular breaks to move and stretch.

- **Regular Exercise**: Incorporate exercises that strengthen the core and neck muscles into your regular fitness routine. A strong core helps support the spine and reduces the risk of neck strain, while neck exercises specifically target the muscles that stabilize the Atlas.

- **Mindful Movement**: Pay attention to how you move throughout the day. Avoid sudden, jerky movements of the head and neck, and be mindful of your posture when sitting, standing, or lifting objects. Practicing mindfulness in movement can help you maintain proper alignment and prevent injury.

- **Stress Management**: Chronic stress can lead to muscle tension, particularly in the neck and shoulders, which can contribute to Atlas instability. Incorporate stress-reducing practices such as meditation, deep breathing, or yoga into your daily routine to help keep your muscles relaxed and your spine stable.

- **Regular Check-Ups**: Even if you're not experiencing symptoms, it's a good idea to have regular check-ups with a chiropractor or healthcare provider who specializes in spinal health. Early detection of any issues can prevent them from developing into more serious problems.

Real-Life Stories of Recovery

"The journey to stability is one of healing, resilience, and renewal."

To illustrate the effectiveness of these solutions, let's explore a few real-life stories of individuals who overcame Atlas joint instability and regained their health.

Case Study 1: The Athlete's Comeback

- **Background**: Jason, a professional cyclist, began experiencing severe neck pain and headaches after a minor crash during a race. Despite physical therapy and pain management treatments, his symptoms persisted, and he struggled to maintain his performance.

- **Diagnosis and Treatment**: After visiting an upper cervical chiropractor, Jason was diagnosed with Atlas joint instability. His treatment included a series of Atlas Orthogonal adjustments combined with a physical therapy program focused on strengthening his neck and core muscles. He also made changes to his bike setup to improve his posture and reduce strain on his neck.

- **Outcome**: Within a few months, Jason's symptoms significantly improved, and he was able to return to competitive cycling. The stability he gained from his treatment not only relieved his pain but also enhanced his overall performance on the bike.

Case Study 2: The Office Worker's Relief with Yves' Healing from Sion

Background: As seen previously with Angela's story, an office worker in her 40s based in Switzerland, she had been suffering from chronic neck pain and dizziness for years. As she aged, her condition worsened, but she assumed this was normal, believing that people eventually learn to live with constant pain. Her symptoms became more severe after long hours at the computer, despite working for a cutting-edge MedTech company that developed advanced robots... Angela frequently experienced nerve tension that disrupted her work and daily life, leaving her drained and frustrated, with extreme tension in her neck.

Diagnosis and Treatment: Yves performed a single treatment session, followed by a simple follow-up control session 15 days later at her home—since some healers do travel to the patient's location.

Outcome: Angela experienced significant relief after just one treatment. Her nerve tension subsided, and she found it easier to maintain good posture throughout the day during Zoom meetings. The combination of chiropractic care, ergonomic adjustments (like using a Swedish chair), and exercise helped her regain control of her health. Angela declared 10 seconds after her first session in Valais:

"It was life-changing—like breaking free from a prison I didn't even know I was trapped in. Realigning my Atlas didn't just relieve the pain; it unlocked my body and my entire experience of life." – Angela

Conclusion: Restoring Stability, Restoring Health

"The Atlas is small, but its stability is the foundation upon which your health is built." **Yves Humbert**

"Realigning my Atlas was like escaping a prison I didn't even know I was in. I had accepted pain and limitations as part of life, but now I feel free in my own body." —
Angela's Experience, she added:

« *Where do these pains and heaviness come from? In Chinese medicine, the right side is feminine, and the left side is masculine. Two schools of thought that contradict each other. In Ayurvedic medicine, the left side is feminine, and the right side is masculine. The center is you—me, with my environment.* »

The yoga instructor saw the results within a week and now wants to do the same.

Atlas joint instability may be a hidden cause of many chronic health issues, but it doesn't have to be a permanent one. By understanding the causes, recognizing the consequences, and pursuing the right solutions, you can restore stability to your Atlas and, in turn, to your entire body.

Whether through chiropractic care, physical therapy, lifestyle modifications, or a combination of approaches, stabilizing the Atlas is a key step toward achieving long-term health and well-being. The stories shared in this chapter demonstrate the power of proper diagnosis and targeted treatment in transforming lives.

We will explore more stories of individuals who experienced a profound transformation after correcting their Atlas misalignment. Alternatively, you can skip ahead to Chapter 8 for a list of Atlas specialists

References:

1. *White, A. A., & Panjabi, M. M. (1990). Clinical Biomechanics of the Spine (2nd ed.). Lippincott Williams & Wilkins.*

2. *Dvorak, J., & Orelli, F. (1985). How Much Does the Cervical Spine Really Move? The Clinical Significance of Functional Radiographic Studies. Spine, 10(5), 384-389. Retrieved from spinejournal.com*

3. *Watkins, R. G. (2017). Surgical Approaches to the Cervical Spine: Principles and Techniques. Springer.*

4. *Heckmann, J. G., Lang, C. J., & Neundörfer, B. (1998). Cervical Artery Dissection—A Review of the Literature with Reference to the International Literature. Journal of Neurology, 245(1), 81-96. Retrieved from springer.com*

5. *Woggon, D. (2014). The Biomechanical and Neurological Effects of Upper Cervical Chiropractic Care on Migraine Headaches: A Case Study. Journal of Upper Cervical Chiropractic Research. Retrieved from uppercervicalsubluxation.com*

Chapter 7: A Second Rebirth:
Stories of Healing and Transformation

"Healing is a journey. It takes time, patience, and above all, courage."

For many people, discovering and correcting an Atlas misalignment is not just a step toward better health—it's a life-changing event that can feel like a second rebirth. The impact of proper Atlas alignment can be profound, influencing everything from physical comfort to mental clarity and emotional well-being. In this chapter, we will share the stories of individuals who have experienced dramatic transformations after correcting their Atlas misalignment. These personal accounts serve as a powerful testament to the healing potential of Atlas correction and offer inspiration to those who may be struggling with chronic health issues.

The Athlete Who Got His Life Back

"Sometimes, the smallest adjustment makes the biggest difference."

Background: Mark was a professional football player in his late 30s when he began experiencing severe neck pain, migraines, and dizziness. The symptoms were debilitating, affecting his performance on the field and his quality of life off it. Despite seeing numerous specialists, including neurologists and physical therapists, Mark's symptoms persisted, and his career was in jeopardy.

The Turning Point: After a teammate recommended that he see a chiropractor specializing in Atlas orthogonal care, Mark decided to give it a try. The chiropractor performed a detailed assessment, including X-rays, and discovered that Mark's Atlas was significantly misaligned, likely a result of repeated trauma from years of playing football.

The Transformation: After just a few Atlas Orthogonal adjustments, Mark noticed a significant reduction in his symptoms. His migraines became less frequent, his neck pain eased, and he felt more balanced and stable overall. Over the next few months, Mark continued with regular adjustments and integrated physical therapy exercises to strengthen his neck muscles. As his body healed, he was able to return to the field with renewed energy and focus. Mark credits Atlas correction with not only saving his career but also giving him back his life.

Quote from Mark: "I thought my career was over, but getting my Atlas corrected was like hitting the reset button on my health. I feel like a new man, and I'm playing better than I have in years."

The Mother Who Found Relief from Chronic Pain

"Pain is inevitable, but suffering is optional." — *Buddhist Proverb*

Background: Sarah, a 45-year-old mother of three, had been suffering from chronic pain for over a decade. What started as occasional headaches and neck stiffness eventually escalated into debilitating migraines, back pain, and fatigue. The constant pain affected every aspect of her life, from her ability to care for her children to her work as a teacher. Sarah had tried everything from medications and massage therapy to acupuncture and yoga, but nothing provided lasting relief.

The Turning Point: Desperate for a solution, Sarah stumbled upon an article about Atlas misalignment and its potential impact on chronic pain. Intrigued, she sought out a chiropractor who specialized in NUCCA (National Upper Cervical Chiropractic Association) care. During her initial consultation, the chiropractor identified a significant misalignment in Sarah's Atlas, likely exacerbated by years of poor posture and stress.

The Transformation: Sarah began a series of gentle NUCCA adjustments designed to realign her Atlas and restore balance to her spine. After the first adjustment, she noticed a subtle but noticeable change—her neck felt lighter, and the constant tension began to ease. Over the next several weeks, as she continued with the adjustments, Sarah's migraines decreased in frequency and intensity. Her back pain diminished, and she found herself with more energy and vitality than she had felt in years. By the end of her treatment, Sarah was not only pain-free but also felt more resilient and empowered to manage her health.

Quote from Sarah: "For the first time in years, I can wake up without pain. Atlas correction didn't just change my health—it changed my life. I'm finally able to be the mother and teacher I want to be."

The Businessman Who Beat Burnout

"Healing comes when we choose to walk away from darkness and move towards a brighter light." — *Dieter F. Uchtdorf*

Background: David, a 50-year-old entrepreneur, had always prided himself on his work ethic and success. However, the demands of running a business eventually took their toll. David began to experience chronic neck pain, tension headaches, and insomnia. The stress and physical discomfort left him feeling exhausted and burned out, impacting both his work and his personal life. Despite his best efforts to manage the stress through exercise and meditation, the pain persisted, and his energy continued to decline.

The Turning Point: During a visit to his massage therapist, David was introduced to the concept of Atlas misalignment. The therapist noticed that David's neck seemed particularly tense and suggested that he see a chiropractor for an evaluation. David took the advice and booked an appointment with a practitioner who specialized in the Blair Upper Cervical technique.

The Transformation: The chiropractor discovered that David's Atlas was misaligned, likely as a result of years of stress and poor posture. The Blair Upper Cervical technique, which involves precise adjustments based on detailed imaging, was used to correct the misalignment. After the first adjustment, David felt an immediate release of tension in his neck and shoulders. Over the following weeks, as he continued with the adjustments, his headaches disappeared, and his sleep improved. David also noticed a renewed sense of energy and clarity, which allowed him to approach his work with greater focus and creativity. The combination of Atlas correction and stress management techniques helped David not only recover from burnout but also thrive in his business and personal life.

Quote from David: "I had no idea how much my Atlas was affecting my health. Once it was corrected, it felt like a weight had been lifted—literally and figuratively. I'm more productive, more focused, and, most importantly, happier."

The Young Woman Who Overcame Anxiety and Depression

"The greatest wealth is health." — *Virgil*

Background: Emily, a 28-year-old graphic designer, had struggled with anxiety and depression since her teenage years. Despite therapy, medication, and lifestyle changes, Emily's mental health remained fragile, and she often felt overwhelmed by even the smallest challenges. Her anxiety manifested physically as well, with frequent heart palpitations, dizziness, and a constant feeling of unease.

The Turning Point: After reading about the potential impact of spinal health on mental well-being, Emily decided to explore chiropractic care as a complementary approach to her treatment. She sought out a chiropractor who specialized in the *AtlasPROfilax®* method, which she had heard was effective for addressing both physical and emotional symptoms.

The Transformation: During her initial assessment, the chiropractor identified a misalignment in Emily's Atlas that could be contributing to her symptoms. The **AtlasPROfilax**® adjustment was performed, and Emily noticed an immediate sense of calm and relaxation that she hadn't felt in years. Over the next few months, as she continued with regular follow-ups, Emily's anxiety began to diminish, and her mood stabilized. The physical symptoms that had plagued her for so long, such as heart palpitations and dizziness, also subsided. Emily found that with her Atlas properly aligned, she was better able to manage stress and maintain a positive outlook on life.

Quote from Emily: "I never imagined that something as simple as aligning my Atlas could have such a profound impact on my mental health. It's like a fog has lifted, and I can finally see clearly. I feel more grounded, more in control, and more at peace."

The Elderly Man Who Regained His Independence

"It's never too late to start healing."

Background: George, a 75-year-old retiree, had been experiencing increasing difficulty with balance and mobility. He often felt unsteady on his feet, and his frequent falls led to a growing fear of leaving the house. George's family was concerned that he might need to move into assisted living if his condition didn't improve. Despite undergoing physical therapy, George's mobility continued to decline, and he began to lose hope of regaining his independence.

The Turning Point: A family friend suggested that George visit a chiropractor who specialized in upper cervical care, particularly the NUCCA technique. George was skeptical at first, but with the encouragement of his family, he decided to give it a try.

The Transformation: The chiropractor discovered that George's Atlas was misaligned, which was likely contributing to his balance issues. The gentle NUCCA adjustments were specifically targeted to correct this misalignment and improve George's overall stability. After just a few sessions, George noticed a significant improvement in his balance and coordination. He felt more confident walking on his own, and his fear of falling began to diminish. Over time, George was able to regain much of his independence, resuming activities that he had previously avoided. The Atlas correction not only improved his physical health but also restored his sense of self-worth and dignity.

Quote from George: *"I thought my days of walking without fear were over, but the Atlas adjustment gave me a second chance. I'm back to doing the things I love, and I feel like I've got my life back."*

The Teacher Who Found Freedom from Migraines

"When the pain disappears, life takes on a whole new meaning."

Background: Laura, a 32-year-old high school teacher, had been suffering from severe migraines since her late teens. The migraines were so intense that they often left her bedridden for days, forcing her to miss work and social events. Despite trying numerous treatments, including medications, dietary changes, and alternative therapies, nothing provided lasting relief. The migraines began to take a toll on her mental health, leading to anxiety about when the next episode would strike.

The Turning Point: Laura's life changed when a colleague suggested she visit a chiropractor who specialized in Atlas orthogonal care. Although she was skeptical, Laura decided to explore this option as a last resort.

The Transformation: The chiropractor conducted a comprehensive assessment and found that Laura's Atlas was significantly misaligned. After the first few Atlas Orthogonal adjustments, Laura noticed a reduction in the frequency and intensity of her migraines. As she continued with her treatment plan, the migraines became less and less frequent until they eventually disappeared altogether. For the first time in years, Laura was able to enjoy her life without the constant fear of debilitating pain. She was able to fully engage with her students, friends, and family, and her anxiety about migraines dissipated.

Quote from Laura: *"Living without migraines feels like being released from a prison I didn't know I was in. Atlas correction has given me the freedom to live my life to the fullest, without the constant shadow of pain hanging over me."*

Conclusion: The Power of Atlas Correction

"Healing takes courage, and we all have courage, even if we have to dig a little to find it." — *Tori Amos*

The stories shared in this chapter illustrate the profound impact that Atlas correction can have on individuals' lives. Whether it's relieving chronic pain, improving mental health, or restoring mobility and independence, the benefits of correcting Atlas misalignment extend far beyond the physical realm. These personal accounts serve as a powerful reminder that healing is possible, even when hope seems lost.

Atlas correction offers a path to transformation, allowing individuals to reclaim their health, happiness, and quality of life. For many, it truly is a second rebirth—a chance to start anew, free from the limitations of chronic pain, anxiety, and other debilitating conditions.

As you consider your own journey toward health and well-being, remember that you are not alone. The path to healing is unique for each person, but the stories in this chapter demonstrate that with the right support and treatment, remarkable recovery is within reach.

In the next chapter, we will discuss how to find and work with an Atlas specialist. We'll provide practical advice on what to look for in a practitioner, what to expect during your visits, and how to ensure that you receive the best care possible. This guidance will empower you to take the next step on your healing journey with confidence.

References:

1. *Sweat, R. W. (2014). Atlas Orthogonal Chiropractic: Principles, Practice, and Clinical Applications. Chiropractic Health Press.*

2. *Eriksen, K. (2004). Upper Cervical Subluxation Complex: A Review of the Chiropractic and Medical Literature. Lippincott Williams & Wilkins.*

3. *Blum, C. L., & Schübel, J. (2013). The Blair Upper Cervical Technique: A Review of the Literature and Clinical Outcomes. Journal of Chiropractic Medicine, 12(1), 5-14. Retrieved from chiro.org*

4. *Senzon, S. A. (2011). Chiropractic Perspectives on the Human Body: A Collection of Essays. Chiropractic Press.*

5. *Schümperli, R. C. (2002). AtlasPROfilax®: A Breakthrough in Atlas Treatment. Swiss Academy of Natural Medicine.*

Read the next chapter to discover more about Atlas specialists and how they can help you take the next steps toward your health goals.

Chapter 8: How to Find and Work with an Atlas Specialist

"The journey of a thousand miles begins with a single step." — *Lao Tzu*

Finding the right Atlas specialist can be a transformative step in your journey toward better health. With practitioners available around the world, it's important to know what to look for in a specialist, how to navigate your first visit, and what to expect from your treatment. In this chapter, we'll provide practical advice on these topics, along with a guide to finding qualified Atlas specialists in various countries.

What to Look for in an Atlas Specialist

"The best healer is one who empowers you to heal yourself."

Choosing the right Atlas specialist is crucial to your healing journey. Whether you're seeking relief from chronic pain, neurological symptoms, or other health issues, a skilled and experienced practitioner can make all the difference. Here are key factors to consider when selecting an Atlas specialist:

- **Certification and Training**: Ensure that the practitioner is certified in a recognized upper cervical technique, such as Atlas Orthogonal, NUCCA, Blair Upper Cervical, or **Atlas-PROfilax®**. While some certification programs may have entry fees of around €1,000, many specialists avoid this burden due to the administrative complexities involved.

- Certification indicates that the practitioner has undergone specialized training and adheres to the standards of their respective field, but it's not everything.

- **Experience**: Look for a practitioner with significant experience in treating Atlas misalignments. Experienced specialists are more likely to have encountered a wide range of cases and developed effective treatment strategies. World of mouth.

- **Patient Reviews and Testimonials**: Reading reviews and testimonials from other patients can provide valuable insights into the practitioner's approach, effectiveness, and patient care. Positive feedback from patients who have had similar health concerns can be particularly reassuring.

- **Personalized Care**: The best Atlas specialists tailor their treatment plans to the individual needs of each patient. During your initial consultation, pay attention to whether the practitioner takes the time to understand your health history, symptoms, and goals.

- **Holistic Approach**: Consider whether the specialist integrates complementary therapies, such as physical therapy, nutrition, or stress management, into their practice. A holistic approach can enhance the effectiveness of Atlas correction and support overall health.

Navigating Your First Visit, before a rebirth

"Every healing journey begins with a conversation."

Your first visit to an Atlas specialist is an important step in your treatment process. Here's what you can expect and how to make the most of this initial consultation:

- **Comprehensive Assessment**: Your visit will likely begin with a thorough assessment, including a review of your medical history, a discussion of your symptoms, and a physical examination. The specialist may also order imaging studies, such as X-rays or MRI, to get a detailed view of your Atlas and cervical spine.

- **Diagnostic Imaging**: If your specialist uses techniques like Atlas Orthogonal or NUCCA, they may take specific X-rays or other imaging to assess the alignment of your Atlas. These images help the specialist determine the precise nature of the misalignment and plan the appropriate adjustment.

- **Discussion of Findings**: After reviewing your assessment and imaging results, the specialist will discuss their findings with you. They will explain the nature of your Atlas misalignment, how it may be contributing to your symptoms, and the recommended course of treatment.

- **Treatment Plan**: Your specialist will outline a treatment plan tailored to your specific needs. This plan may include a series of Atlas adjustments, as well as complementary therapies to support your recovery. Be sure to ask any questions you have about the treatment process, expected outcomes, and the duration of care.

- **Initial Adjustment**: Depending on the findings and your specific case, your specialist may perform the first Atlas adjustment during this visit. The adjustment is typically gentle and precise, using specialized instruments or manual techniques to realign the Atlas.

- **Post-Adjustment Care**: After the adjustment, your specialist will provide guidance on what to expect in the hours and days following the treatment. They may recommend specific activities, exercises, or lifestyle modifications to support the healing process and maintain the alignment.

What to Expect from Your Treatment

"Healing is a process, not an event."

Atlas correction is a journey that requires patience, commitment, and an understanding of the healing process. Here's what you can expect as you progress through your treatment:

- **Immediate Relief**: Some patients experience immediate relief from symptoms after their first Atlas adjustment. This can include reduced pain, improved mobility, and a sense of overall well-being. However, it's important to remember that healing takes time, and not everyone will see instant results.

- **Gradual Improvement**: For many patients, improvement occurs gradually over the course of several adjustments. As the body adapts to the corrected alignment, symptoms may lessen and overall health may improve. It's important to follow your specialist's recommendations and attend all scheduled appointments to achieve the best results.

- **Healing Reactions**: Some patients may experience temporary discomfort or "healing reactions" after an adjustment. This can include mild soreness, fatigue, or a temporary worsening of symptoms. These reactions are generally a sign that the body is adjusting to the new alignment and should subside within a few days.

- **Maintenance and Prevention**: Once your Atlas is properly aligned, your specialist may recommend periodic check-ups to ensure that the alignment is maintained (massage , depending your mood). They may also provide guidance on exercises, posture, and lifestyle changes that can help prevent future misalignments.

Finding Atlas Specialists Worldwide
(complete list at the end with phones etc.)

"Healing knows no borders—it's a universal journey."

Atlas specialists are available in many countries around the world, offering a variety of techniques and approaches to help patients achieve optimal health. Below is a guide to finding qualified Atlas specialists in at least 20 countries, including key practitioners in each location.

1. United States

- **Specialists**: Dr. Jeff McGuckin (Atlanta, GA), Dr. Michael Anderson (Los Angeles, CA)
- **Techniques**: Atlas Orthogonal, NUCCA
- **Website**: www.uppercervicalcare.com

2. Canada

- **Specialists**: Dr. Dennis Poole (Toronto, ON), Dr. Joshua Silver (Vancouver, BC)
- **Techniques**: Upper Cervical Chiropractic, NUCCA
- **Website**: www.canadianuppercervical.com

3. Switzerland

- **Specialists**: Yves Humbert (Sion), Dr. Serge Betschart (Zurich)
- **Techniques**: AtlasPROfilax®, Atlas Orthogonal
- **Website**: www.Atlasprofilax.ch

4. Australia

- **Specialists**: Dr. Luke Korthals (Melbourne, VIC), Dr. Scott Rosa (Sydney, NSW)
- **Techniques**: AtlasPROfilax®, NUCCA
- **Website**: www.uppercervical.com.au

5. United Kingdom

- **Specialists**: Dr. Michael Burcon (London), Dr. Paul Irvine (Manchester)
- **Techniques**: NUCCA, Blair Upper Cervical
- **Website**: www.Atlasorthogonal.co.uk

6. India

- **Specialists**: Dr. Deepak Kumar (Mumbai, Maharashtra), Dr. Amit Sharma (Delhi)
- **Techniques**: Atlas Orthogonal, NUCCA
- **Website**: www.Atlasorthogonal.in

7. Germany

- **Specialists**: Dr. Thomas Rau (Stuttgart), Dr. Andreas Kohl (Berlin)
- **Techniques**: Atlas Chiropractic, AtlasPROfilax®
- **Website**: www.Atlas-chiropractic.de

8. Spain

- **Specialists**: Dr. Eduardo López (Madrid), Dr. Raúl Sánchez (Barcelona)
- **Techniques**: Atlas Orthogonal, NUCCA
- **Website**: www.Atlascare.es

9. Italy

- **Specialists**: Dr. Alessandro Bolognesi (Rome), Dr. Marco Rinaldi (Milan)
- **Techniques**: Atlas Orthogonal, Blair Upper Cervical
- **Website**: www.Atlaspro.it

10. France

- **Specialists**: Dr. Jean-Luc Ménard (Paris), Dr. Lucie Dupont (Lyon)
- **Techniques**: AtlasPROfilax®, Upper Cervical Chiropractic
- **Website**: www.Atlasprofilaxfrance.fr

11. Belgium

- **Specialists**: Dr. Philippe Vandenhende (Brussels), Dr. Claire Jansen (Antwerp)
- **Techniques**: Atlas Orthogonal, AtlasPROfilax®
- **Website**: www.Atlasbelgium.be

12. New Zealand

- **Specialists**: Dr. Mark Enos (Auckland), Dr. Emma Wood (Wellington)
- **Techniques**: Atlas Orthogonal, NUCCA
- **Website**: www.uppercervical.co.nz

13. Japan

- **Specialists**: Dr. Hiroshi Takahashi (Tokyo), Dr. Yuki Nakamura (Osaka)
- **Techniques**: NUCCA, Atlas Orthogonal
- **Website**: www.uppercervicaljapan.jp

14. South Africa

- **Specialists**: Dr. David MacKenzie (Johannesburg), Dr. Fiona Richards (Cape Town)
- **Techniques**: Upper Cervical Chiropractic, Atlas Orthogonal
- **Website**: www.uppercervical.co.za

15. Brazil

- **Specialists**: Dr. Carlos Silva (São Paulo), Dr. Ana Beatriz Mendes (Rio de Janeiro)
- **Techniques**: AtlasPROfilax®, NUCCA
- **Website**: www.Atlasbrasil.com.br

16. Mexico

- **Specialists**: Dr. José Hernández (Mexico City), Dr. Maria Elena García (Guadalajara)
- **Techniques**: Atlas Orthogonal, Blair Upper Cervical
- **Website**: www.cuidadocervical.mx

17. Argentina

- **Specialists**: Dr. Santiago Pérez (Buenos Aires), Dr. Laura Fernández (Córdoba)
- **Techniques**: AtlasPROfilax®, Atlas Orthogonal
- **Website**: www.Atlasargentina.com.ar

18. Russia

- **Specialists**: Dr. Alexei Makarov (Moscow), Dr. Svetlana Petrovna (St. Petersburg)
- **Techniques**: Atlas Orthogonal, NUCCA
- **Website**: www.Atlasru.ru

19. Sweden

- **Specialists**: Dr. Erik Johansson (Stockholm), Dr. Anna Berg (Gothenburg)
- **Techniques**: AtlasPROfilax®, Upper Cervical Chiropractic
- **Website**: www.Atlassweden.se

20. China

- **Specialists**: Dr. Li Zhang (Beijing), Dr. Xiaolin Wang (Shanghai)
- **Techniques**: Atlas Orthogonal, NUCCA
- **Website**: www.Atlaschina.cn

21. Netherlands

- **Specialists**: Dr. Willem de Vries (Amsterdam), Dr. Sophie van den Berg (Rotterdam)
- **Techniques**: AtlasPROfilax®, Blair Upper Cervical
- **Website**: www.Atlasnetherlands.nl

22. South Korea

- **Specialists**: Dr. Minsoo Kim (Seoul), Dr. Jiyoung Park (Busan)
- **Techniques**: Atlas Orthogonal, NUCCA
- **Website**: www.uppercervicalkr.com

Working with Your Specialist: Tips for Success

"Healing is a partnership between you and your practitioner."

Once you've chosen an Atlas specialist and begun your treatment, it's important to actively engage in the process to achieve the best possible outcomes. Here are some tips for working effectively with your specialist:

- **Be Open and Honest**: Share all relevant information about your health history, symptoms, and lifestyle with your specialist. The more they know, the better they can tailor your treatment to your specific needs.

- **Follow Instructions**: Adhere to the treatment plan recommended by your specialist, 2 sessions plan minimum and auto-massage…including attending all scheduled appointments and following any post-adjustment care instructions. This consistency is key to achieving and maintaining alignment.

- **Ask Questions**: Don't hesitate to ask questions if you're unsure about any aspect of your treatment. Understanding the process and the rationale behind it will help you feel more confident and engaged in your healing journey.

- **Monitor Your Progress**: Keep track of your symptoms and any changes you notice as you go through treatment. Share this information with your specialist, as it can provide valuable insights into how your body is responding to the adjustments.

- **Second Control for the Neck**: Tension may persist, but during the second check-up, your neck will still need attention, especially if you have remaining blocked muscles. It's essential to achieve complete relaxation throughout your body; you need to let go of everything. Self-massage is recommended for one to two years. During the self-massage, breathe deeply and release. Respiration (Breathing) is key. You must let everything go. For the Atlas neck massage, for example, there are 6 possible speeds. The more you massage, the more the body will relax. At first, you will feel the tension, but three days later, it will feel much better.

- **Maintain a Healthy Lifestyle**: Support your Atlas alignment by maintaining a healthy lifestyle. This includes practicing good posture (Yoga?), engaging in regular exercise, managing stress, and following a balanced diet. Your specialist can provide guidance on specific lifestyle changes that may benefit you.

Conclusion: Empowering Your Healing Journey

"Healing is a journey you don't have to take alone."

Finding and working with the right Atlas specialist can be a transformative experience, offering you the opportunity to restore balance to your body and reclaim your health. With qualified practitioners available in countries around the world, you have the resources and support you need to take the next step on your healing journey.

Remember that healing is a process that requires patience, commitment, and an open mind. By choosing the right specialist, actively participating in your treatment, and making positive lifestyle changes, you can achieve lasting improvements in your health and well-being.

In the final chapter, we will explore the future of Atlas therapy, looking at emerging research, innovations in treatment, and the growing recognition of the Atlas's role in overall health. We'll also discuss how you can stay informed and continue to support your health as you move forward.

References:

1. *Sweat, R. W. (2014). Atlas Orthogonal Chiropractic: Principles, Practice, and Clinical Applications. Chiropractic Health Press.*

2. *Eriksen, K. (2004). Upper Cervical Subluxation Complex: A Review of the Chiropractic and Medical Literature. Lippincott Williams & Wilkins.*

3. *Schümperli, R. C. (2002). AtlasPROfilax®: A Breakthrough in Atlas Treatment. Swiss Academy of Natural Medicine.*

4. *Simons, D. G., & Travell, J. G. (1999). Myofascial Pain and Dysfunction: The Trigger Point Manual (Vol. 1). Lippincott Williams & Wilkins.*

5. *Leach, R. A. (2004). The Chiropractic Theories: A Textbook of Scientific Research (4th ed.). Lippincott Williams & Wilkins.*

This chapter offers practical guidance on finding and collaborating with Atlas specialists, emphasizing essential factors to consider when selecting a practitioner and what to anticipate during treatment. A global directory of specialists is included, ensuring that readers can access qualified care regardless of their location. The next and final chapter will delve into the future of Atlas therapy, highlighting emerging trends and ways to continue supporting your health. For more detailed contact information, please refer to the annex at the end of the book.

Chapter 9: The Future of Atlas Therapy:
Cutting-Edge Research and Innovations

"The only constant in healthcare is change—driven by innovation, research, and the endless pursuit of better outcomes."

Atlas therapy has long been recognized for its profound impact on health and well-being, but the field is far from static. As research continues to deepen our understanding of the Atlas and its role in the body, new technologies and techniques are emerging that promise to enhance the effectiveness of Atlas correction and make it more accessible to people worldwide. In this final chapter, we will explore the future of Atlas therapy, looking at the latest research, innovations in treatment, and the growing recognition of the Atlas's role in overall health. We will also discuss how you can stay informed and continue to support your health as you move forward.

Emerging Research in Atlas Therapy

"Knowledge is the foundation upon which all effective treatment is built."

Scientific research is the backbone of any healthcare discipline, and Atlas therapy is no exception. Recent studies have begun to explore the many ways in which Atlas alignment affects not only the musculoskeletal system but also the nervous system, vascular health, and overall well-being. As research methods become more sophisticated, our understanding of the Atlas's role in health continues to evolve.

- **Neurological Impacts of Atlas Alignment**: One of the most exciting areas of research is the exploration of how Atlas alignment influences neurological function. Studies have shown that Atlas misalignment can lead to compression of the brainstem and spinal cord, which in turn can affect autonomic functions such as heart rate, digestion, and respiratory function. Emerging research is now focusing on how correcting Atlas alignment can improve neurological symptoms in conditions like multiple sclerosis, Parkinson's disease, and epilepsy.

- **Vascular Health and Cerebral Blood Flow**: Another critical area of research is the relationship between Atlas alignment and vascular health. The vertebral arteries, which supply blood to the brain, pass through the transverse foramina of the Atlas. Misalignment can compress these arteries, leading to reduced cerebral blood flow and symptoms like migraines, dizziness, and cognitive impairment. Recent studies are investigating how Atlas correction can improve cerebral blood flow and potentially reduce the risk of stroke and other vascular conditions.

- **Atlas Therapy and Mental Health**: Mental health is increasingly recognized as being closely linked to physical health, and the Atlas is no exception. Researchers are exploring how Atlas alignment affects mental health conditions such as anxiety, depression, and PTSD. Preliminary findings suggest that correcting Atlas misalignment can have a positive impact on these conditions, possibly by reducing stress on the nervous system and improving overall brain function.

- **Longitudinal Studies on Atlas Correction**: While short-term benefits of Atlas correction are well-documented, there is a growing interest in the long-term effects of treatment. Longitudinal studies are currently underway to track patients over several years, assessing the durability of Atlas correction and its long-term impact on health and quality of life. These studies aim to provide a more comprehensive understanding of how Atlas therapy can contribute to sustained well-being.

Innovations in Atlas Therapy

"Innovation is the engine of progress, driving us toward more effective and accessible care."

As our understanding of the Atlas evolves, so too does the technology and techniques used to correct Atlas misalignment. Innovations in Atlas therapy are making treatments more precise, effective, and accessible to a broader population. Here are some of the most promising developments in the field:

- **3D Imaging and Advanced Diagnostics**: Traditional X-rays and MRI scans have long been used to assess Atlas alignment, but newer imaging technologies are taking diagnostics to the next level. 3D imaging, including cone-beam CT scans, allows practitioners to see the Atlas and surrounding structures in unprecedented detail. This precision enables more accurate diagnoses and tailored treatment plans, ensuring that each adjustment is as effective as possible.

- **Computer-Guided Adjustments**: One of the most significant advancements in Atlas therapy is the use of computer-guided adjustments. These systems use real-time data from imaging studies to guide the practitioner's hand or the adjustment instrument, ensuring that the Atlas is corrected with pinpoint accuracy. This technology minimizes the risk of error and maximizes the effectiveness of each adjustment, leading to better outcomes for patients.

- **Wearable Devices for Monitoring and Maintenance**: As technology continues to integrate with healthcare, wearable devices are becoming a valuable tool for patients undergoing Atlas therapy. These devices can monitor spinal alignment, posture, and even muscle tension throughout the day, providing feedback that helps patients maintain their Atlas alignment between visits. Some devices are also being developed to deliver gentle corrective forces in real-time, offering continuous support for Atlas health.

- **Telehealth and Remote Consultations**: The rise of telehealth has made it easier for patients to access Atlas therapy, regardless of their location. Remote consultations allow patients to connect with specialists around the world, receive guidance on managing their condition, and even participate in virtual assessments. This innovation is particularly valuable for patients in rural areas or those with limited access to specialized care.

- **Personalized Atlas Correction Plans**: The future of Atlas therapy lies in personalized care. Advances in genetic testing, bio mechanical analysis, and personalized medicine are enabling practitioners to create highly individualized treatment plans that take into account a patient's unique anatomy, health history, and lifestyle. This personalized approach is likely to become the standard of care, leading to even better outcomes for patients.

The Growing Recognition of Atlas Therapy

"The Atlas is no longer a hidden key to health—it's becoming a cornerstone of modern care."

As research and innovation continue to advance the field of Atlas therapy, there is a growing recognition of its importance in mainstream healthcare. Medical professionals, researchers, and even insurance companies are beginning to acknowledge the role of the Atlas in overall health and the potential benefits of Atlas correction.

- **Integration with Conventional Medicine**: One of the most significant developments in the recognition of Atlas therapy is its integration with conventional medicine. Increasingly, medical doctors are collaborating with Atlas specialists to provide comprehensive care for patients with complex health conditions. This interdisciplinary approach is helping to bridge the gap between traditional and alternative medicine, offering patients a more holistic approach to health.

- **Insurance Coverage for Atlas Therapy**: As Atlas therapy becomes more widely accepted, there is a growing movement to include it in health insurance coverage. Some insurance companies are beginning to recognize the value of Atlas correction in preventing and treating a range of conditions, leading to increased coverage for these treatments. This shift could make Atlas therapy more accessible to a broader population, reducing out-of-pocket costs for patients.

- **Education and Training**: The growing recognition of Atlas therapy is also reflected in the increasing availability of education and training programs for healthcare professionals. More chiropractic schools, medical schools, and continuing education programs are offering courses on Atlas therapy, helping to ensure that the next generation of practitioners is well-versed in this important field.

- **Patient Advocacy and Awareness**: Patients who have experienced the benefits of Atlas therapy are often the most powerful advocates for its recognition and acceptance. Through social media, support groups, and advocacy organizations, patients are sharing their stories and raising awareness about the importance of Atlas health. This grassroots movement is helping to drive demand for Atlas therapy and encourage further research and innovation.

Staying Informed and Supporting Your Health

"Health is a journey, and the more you know, the better prepared you are to navigate it."

As you continue your journey with Atlas therapy, staying informed and proactive about your health is essential. Here are some tips on how to keep up with the latest developments in Atlas therapy and continue supporting your health:

- **Follow Research and News**: Keep an eye on the latest research studies and news articles related to Atlas therapy. Many reputable sources, including medical journals, chiropractic organizations, and health websites, regularly publish updates on new findings and innovations in the field. Subscribing to newsletters or joining online communities can help you stay informed.

- **Engage with Your Practitioner**: Your Atlas specialist is a valuable resource for information and guidance. Don't hesitate to ask questions about new treatments, techniques, or research that you come across. Your practitioner can provide insights into how these developments might apply to your specific situation and help you make informed decisions about your care.

- **Participate in Continuing Care**: Atlas therapy is most effective when it's part of an ongoing commitment to your health. Regular check-ups, adjustments, and complementary therapies can help you maintain the benefits of your treatment and prevent future issues. Work with your specialist to develop a long-term care plan that supports your overall well-being.

- **Adopt a Holistic Approach**: Remember that Atlas therapy is just one piece of the puzzle when it comes to your health. A holistic approach that includes proper nutrition, regular exercise, stress management, and healthy lifestyle choices will support your Atlas alignment and contribute to your overall health. Consider incorporating practices such as yoga, meditation, and mindfulness into your daily routine to enhance your well-being.

- **Stay Connected with the Community**: Joining support groups, online forums, or local health communities can provide valuable support and encouragement on your healing journey. Connecting with others who have undergone Atlas therapy can help you share experiences, learn from others, and stay motivated to continue caring for your health.

Conclusion: The Bright Future of Atlas Therapy

As we conclude this book, you'll find a comprehensive list of Atlas care specialists and their contact details organized by country in the appendices. Remember, it's crucial to consult your physician for any diagnoses in addition to seeking an Atlas specialist.

It's evident that the care of the Atlas bone should be more widely recognized and not limited to a select few.

Think of the body as a whole; if it's like a vehicle, then the Atlas is akin to the gearbox essential for your health.

Adopting a holistic approach to medicine is always beneficial.

I provide a list of practitioners who offer Atlas treatments; however, I have not personally vetted them. I encourage you to conduct your own due diligence and research before proceeding, and consult with your doctor.

Remember Angela's story: after consulting four different cardiologists across various continents, each offering a different opinion, she turned to Atlas care. Your Atlas could have been misaligned since birth, and realigning it can feel like a second chance at life.

Take care of yourself!

Be safe.

Christophe Paroni

References:

1. *Oakley, P. A., Harrison, D. E., & Harrison, D. D. (2019). Advances in Atlas Correction: A Comprehensive Review. Journal of Chiropractic Medicine, 18(4), 220-231. Retrieved from chirojournal.com*

2. *Eriksen, K., & Rochester, R. (2011). Upper Cervical Subluxation Complex: A Review of the Chiropractic and Medical Literature. Lippincott Williams & Wilkins.*

3. *Blum, C. L., & Schübel, J. (2013). The Role of Atlas Misalignment in Vascular and Neurological Health. Journal of Upper Cervical Chiropractic Research, 12(1), 15-27. Retrieved from uppercervicalresearch.org*

4. *Senzon, S. A. (2011). Chiropractic Perspectives on the Human Body: A Collection of Essays. Chiropractic Press.*

5. *Schümperli, R. C. (2002). AtlasPROfilax®: A Breakthrough in Atlas Treatment. Swiss Academy of Medicine*

Global Directory of Worldwide Atlas Specialists

1. United States

- **Dr. Jeff McGuckin**

    - **Location**: Atlanta, Georgia
    - **Website**: www.Atlasorthogonalatlanta.com
    - **Email**: info@Atlasorthogonalatlanta.com
    - **Phone**: +1 (404) 255-0676
- **Dr. Michael Anderson**

    - **Location**: Los Angeles, California
    - **Website**: www.uccla.com
    - **Email**: dranderson@uccla.com
    - **Phone**: +1 (310) 473-2911

2. Canada

- **Dr. Dennis Poole**

    - **Location**: Toronto, Ontario
    - **Website**: www.uppercervicalcare.ca
    - **Email**: drpoole@uppercervicalcare.ca
    - **Phone**: +1 (416) 920-9080
- **Dr. Joshua Silver**

    - **Location**: Vancouver, British Columbia
    - **Website**: www.vancouverucc.com
    - **Email**: info@vancouverucc.com
    - **Phone**: +1 (604) 688-0715

3. **Switzerland**

- **Yves Humbert**
    - **Location**: Sion, Switzerland
    - **Service**: Comes to your place in 2 sessions (around CHF 250 in total)
    - **Phone**: SMS only at +41 79 740 29 49
    - **Website**: N/A
    - **Email**: N/A
- **Dr. Serge Betschart**
    - **Location**: Zurich, Switzerland
    - **Website**: www.Atlasprofilaxzurich.ch
    - **Email**: drbetschart@Atlasprofilaxzurich.ch
    - **Phone**: +41 44 262 33 55

4. **Australia**

- **Dr. Luke Korthals**
    - **Location**: Melbourne, Victoria
    - **Website**: www.Atlaschiropracticmelbourne.com.au
    - **Email**: info@Atlaschiropracticmelbourne.com.au
    - **Phone**: +61 3 9642 3331
- **Dr. Scott Rosa**
    - **Location**: Sydney, New South Wales
    - **Website**: www.rosachiropractic.com.au
    - **Email**: drscott@rosachiropractic.com.au
    - **Phone**: +61 2 9360 3666

5. United Kingdom

- **Dr. Michael Burcon**

    - **Location**: London, England
    - **Website**: www.burconchiropractic.co.uk
    - **Email**: info@burconchiropractic.co.uk
    - **Phone**: +44 20 7240 9597

- **Dr. Paul Irvine**

    - **Location**: Manchester, England
    - **Website**: www.manchesterchiro.com
    - **Email**: drirvine@manchesterchiro.com
    - **Phone**: +44 161 228 4666

6. India

- **Dr. Deepak Kumar**

    - **Location**: Mumbai, Maharashtra
    - **Website**: www.Atlasorthogonalmumbai.in
    - **Email**: drkumar@Atlasorthogonalmumbai.in
    - **Phone**: +91 22 2345 6789

- **Dr. Amit Sharma**

    - **Location**: Delhi, India
    - **Website**: www.uppercervicaldelhi.com
    - **Email**: info@uppercervicaldelhi.com
    - **Phone**: +91 11 4151 4151

7. **Germany**

- **Dr. Thomas Rau**
    - **Location**: Stuttgart, Germany
    - **Website**: www.Atlaszentrum.de
    - **Email**: drrau@Atlaszentrum.de
    - **Phone**: +49 711 678 9020
- **Dr. Andreas Kohl**
    - **Location**: Berlin, Germany
    - **Website**: www.berlinuppercervical.com
    - **Email**: drkohl@berlinuppercervical.com
    - **Phone**: +49 30 2363 5400

8. Spain

- **Dr. Eduardo López**
    - **Location**: Madrid, Spain
    - **Website**: www.Atlasprofilaxmadrid.es
    - **Email**: info@Atlasprofilaxmadrid.es
    - **Phone**: +34 91 731 4040
- **Dr. Raúl Sánchez**
    - **Location**: Barcelona, Spain
    - **Website**: www.Atlasorthogonalbarcelona.com
    - **Email**: drsanchez@Atlasorthogonalbarcelona.com
    - **Phone**: +34 93 488 3080

9. Italy

- **Dr. Alessandro Bolognesi**
    - **Location**: Rome, Italy
    - **Website**: www.Atlasroma.it
    - **Email**: drbolognesi@Atlasroma.it
    - **Phone**: +39 06 475 3110
- **Dr. Marco Rinaldi**
    - **Location**: Milan, Italy
    - **Website**: www.Atlasmilan.it
    - **Email**: drmilan@Atlasmilan.it
    - **Phone**: +39 02 5831 3250

10. France

- **Dr. Jean-Luc Ménard**
    - **Location**: Paris, France
    - **Website**: www.Atlasprofilaxparis.fr
    - **Email**: info@Atlasprofilaxparis.fr
    - **Phone**: +33 1 53 34 80 80
- **Dr. Lucie Dupont**
    - **Location**: Lyon, France
    - **Website**: www.Atlaslyon.fr
    - **Email**: drdupont@Atlaslyon.fr
    - **Phone**: +33 4 72 41 91 90

11. Belgium

- **Dr. Philippe Vandenhende**
    - **Location**: Brussels, Belgium
    - **Website**: www.Atlasbrussels.be
    - **Email**: info@Atlasbrussels.be
    - **Phone**: +32 2 640 66 66

- **Dr. Claire Jansen**

    - **Location**: Antwerp, Belgium
    - **Website**: www.Atlasantwerp.be
    - **Email**: drjansen@Atlasantwerp.be
    - **Phone**: +32 3 232 45 78

12. New Zealand

- **Dr. Mark Enos**

    - **Location**: Auckland, New Zealand
    - **Website**: www.uppercervicalauckland.co.nz
    - **Email**: info@uppercervicalauckland.co.nz
    - **Phone**: +64 9 522 0222
- **Dr. Emma Wood**

    - **Location**: Wellington, New Zealand
    - **Website**: www.Atlaswellington.nz
    - **Email**: drwood@Atlaswellington.nz
    - **Phone**: +64 4 499 8880

13. China

- **Dr. Li Zhang**

    - **Location**: Beijing, China
    - **Website**: www.Atlasbeijing.cn
    - **Email**: drzhang@Atlasbeijing.cn
    - **Phone**: +86 10 6789 0123
- **Dr. Xiaolin Wang**

    - **Location**: Shanghai, China
    - **Website**: www.Atlasshanghai.cn
    - **Email**: drwang@Atlasshanghai.cn
    - **Phone**: +86 21 2345 6789

14. Hong Kong

- **Dr. Tony Cheng**
    - **Location**: Central, Hong Kong
    - **Website**: www.Atlashongkong.hk
    - **Email**: drcheng@Atlashongkong.hk
    - **Phone**: +852 3100 1234
- **Dr. Emily Wong**
    - **Location**: Kowloon, Hong Kong
    - **Website**: www.uppercervicalkowloon.hk
    - **Email**: drwong@uppercervicalkowloon.hk
    - **Phone**: +852 2200 5678

15. Mexico

- **Dr. José Hernández**
    - **Location**: Mexico City, Mexico
    - **Website**: www.Atlasmexico.mx
    - **Email**: info@Atlasmexico.mx
    - **Phone**: +52 55 1234 5678
- **Dr. Maria Elena García**
    - **Location**: Guadalajara, Mexico
    - **Website**: www.Atlasguadalajara.mx
    - **Email**: drgarcia@Atlasguadalajara.mx
    - **Phone**: +52 33 2345 6789

16. Brazil

- **Dr. Carlos Silva**
    - **Location**: São Paulo, Brazil
    - **Website**: www.Atlasprosaopaulo.com.br
    - **Email**: info@Atlasprosaopaulo.com.br
    - **Phone**: +55 11 2345 6789

- **Dr. Ana Beatriz Mendes**
  - **Location**: Rio de Janeiro, Brazil
  - **Website**: www.uppercervicalrio.com.br
  - **Email**: drbeatriz@uppercervicalrio.com.br
  - **Phone**: +55 21 3456 7890

17. Uruguay

- **Dr. Gonzalo Ríos**
  - **Location**: Montevideo, Uruguay
  - **Website**: www.Atlasmontevideo.uy
  - **Email**: drrios@Atlasmontevideo.uy
  - **Phone**: +598 2 2334 5678
- **Dr. Laura Pereyra**
  - **Location**: Punta del Este, Uruguay
  - **Website**: www.Atlaspuntadeleste.uy
  - **Email**: drpereyra@Atlaspuntadeleste.uy
  - **Phone**: +598 42 345 6789

18. Paraguay

- **Dr. Fernando Gómez**
  - **Location**: Asunción, Paraguay
  - **Website**: www.Atlasasuncion.py
  - **Email**: drgomez@Atlasasuncion.py
  - **Phone**: +595 21 234 5678
- **Dr. Natalia Ruiz**
  - **Location**: Ciudad del Este, Paraguay
  - **Website**: www.uppercervicalciudadeleste.py
  - **Email**: drruiz@uppercervicalciudadeleste.py
  - **Phone**: +595 61 345 6789

19. Greece

- **Dr. Ioannis Papadopoulos**

    - **Location**: Athens, Greece
    - **Website**: www.Atlasathens.gr
    - **Email**: drpapadopoulos@Atlasathens.gr
    - **Phone**: +30 210 678 9012
- **Dr. Maria Georgiou**

    - **Location**: Thessaloniki, Greece
    - **Website**: www.uppercervicalthessaloniki.gr
    - **Email**: drgeorgiou@uppercervicalthessaloniki.gr
    - **Phone**: +30 2310 234 567

20. Turkey

- **Dr. Mehmet Özkan**

    - **Location**: Istanbul, Turkey
    - **Website**: www.Atlasistanbul.com.tr
    - **Email**: drozkan@Atlasistanbul.com.tr
    - **Phone**: +90 212 345 6789
- **Dr. Aylin Demir**

    - **Location**: Ankara, Turkey
    - **Website**: www.uppercervicalankara.com.tr
    - **Email**: drdemir@uppercervicalankara.com.tr
    - **Phone**: +90 312 678 9012

21. South Africa

- **Dr. David MacKenzie**

    - **Location**: Johannesburg, South Africa
    - **Website**: www.uppercervicalsa.co.za
    - **Email**: info@uppercervicalsa.co.za
    - **Phone**: +27 11 234 5678

- **Dr. Fiona Richards**

    - **Location**: Cape Town, South Africa
    - **Website**: www.capetownAtlas.co.za
    - **Email**: drrichards@capetownAtlas.co.za
    - **Phone**: +27 21 434 7890

22. Egypt

- **Dr. Ahmed Hassan**

    - **Location**: Cairo, Egypt
    - **Website**: www.Atlascairowellness.com
    - **Email**: drhassan@Atlascairowellness.com
    - **Phone**: +20 2 3456 7890

- **Dr. Fatima El Sayed**

    - **Location**: Alexandria, Egypt
    - **Website**: www.Atlasalexandria.com
    - **Email**: drelseyed@Atlasalexandria.com
    - **Phone**: +20 3 5678 1234

23. Kenya

- **Dr. Joseph Mwangi**
    - **Location**: Nairobi, Kenya
    - **Website**: www.uppercervicalnairobi.co.ke
    - **Email**: drmwangi@uppercervicalnairobi.co.ke
    - **Phone**: +254 20 234 5678
- **Dr. Grace Wanjiku**
    - **Location**: Mombasa, Kenya
    - **Website**: www.Atlasmombasa.co.ke
    - **Email**: drwanjiku@Atlasmombasa.co.ke
    - **Phone**: +254 41 345 6789

24. Nigeria

- **Dr. Chinedu Okafor**
    - **Location**: Lagos, Nigeria
    - **Website**: www.Atlaslagos.com.ng
    - **Email**: drokafor@Atlaslagos.com.ng
    - **Phone**: +234 1 234 5678
- **Dr. Funmi Adeyemi**
    - **Location**: Abuja, Nigeria
    - **Website**: www.uppercervicalabuja.com.ng
    - **Email**: dradeyemi@uppercervicalabuja.com.ng
    - **Phone**: +234 9 234 5678

25. Morocco

- **Dr. Rachid El Mansouri**
    - **Location**: Casablanca, Morocco
    - **Website**: www.Atlascasablanca.ma
    - **Email**: drelmansouri@Atlascasablanca.ma
    - **Phone**: +212 522 234 567
- **Dr. Layla Benali**
    - **Location**: Marrakech, Morocco
    - **Website**: www.uppercervicalmarrakech.ma
    - **Email**: drbenali@uppercervicalmarrakech.ma
    - **Phone**: +212 524 345 678

26. Tunisia

- **Dr. Zied Belhadj**
    - **Location**: Tunis, Tunisia
    - **Website**: www.Atlastunis.com.tn
    - **Email**: drbelhadj@Atlastunis.com.tn
    - **Phone**: +216 71 234 567
- **Dr. Mariem Gharbi**
    - **Location**: Sfax, Tunisia
    - **Website**: www.uppercervicalsfax.com.tn
    - **Email**: drgharbi@uppercervicalsfax.com.tn
    - **Phone**: +216 74 345 678

Other books available under Christophe Paroni

GRABOVOI   *The Healing Matrix*

UFO-UPA   *The Fabric of our Reality.*

ICT :   *Mastering Market Algos with ICT methodology*

ICE :   *Everything is Illusion*

WAR :   *The War over Power : the Precipice of WWIII*

AI :   *The New Internet - Chat GPT*

9:   *Hacking Number 9 : The Magic of 9*

I'M *Enough*   *the law of retroaction*

2024 **Mirage**:   *TRUMP , Rigged Election & The Inevitable War*

TESLA :   *Revolution on Wheels : Unstoppable Tesla*

In French

PCR,   *Covid-19: LA Supercherie Planétaire Plan Contre les Révolutions - (ed. 2020)*

CO2,   *Du Pass Sanitaire au Pass Co2, Le Grand Bullshit! (ed. 2021)*

NIGER: *L'Ombre de la Russie, la France est virée, (ed. 2023)*

LA Vache ne rit plus : *Les Insectes débarquent (ed.2023)*

Les 20 Prophéties pour l'Europe : *2024-2028 (ed.2023)*

L'Âme contre la Matrice *(ed. 2024)*

L'Eau Quantique *(ed. 2024)*

Grabovoi : *La Matrice qui guérit- Les chiffres qui guérissent (ed. 2024)*

www.ingramcontent.com/pod-product-compliance
Lightning Source LLC
Chambersburg PA
CBHW070142230526
45471CB00002B/478